The HERO GUIDE TO HEALTH:
Health Assessment & Obesity Prevention

Debbie Kantor, BSN, MSN

&

Lt. Sherrin Whiteman

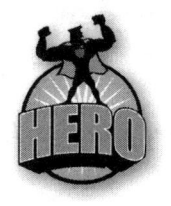

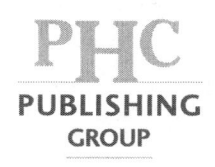

PHC PUBLISHING GROUP

PHC Publishing Group is an imprint of:
PESI HealthCare
A Non-profit Organization
Continuing Education Provider since 1979

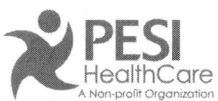

Eau Claire, Wisconsin © 2012

Copyright © 2012

Published by PHC Publishing Group, an imprint of:

PESI HealthCare
200 Spring Street
Eau Claire, WI 54702

ISBN: 978-1-937661-09-0

All rights reserved. No part of the material protected by this copyright may be reproduced or utilized in any form, electronic or mechanical, including photocopying, recording, or by any information storage and retrieval system, without written permission from the copyright owner.

As of press time, the URLs displayed in this publication link or refer to existing websites on the Internet. PESI HealthCare is not responsible for, and should not be deemed to endorse or recommend, any website other than its own or any content available on the internet (including without limitation at any website, blog page, information page) that is not created by PESI HealthCare or PHC Publishing Group.

PESI HealthCare strives to obtain knowledgeable authors and faculty for its publications and seminars. The clinical recommendations contained herein are the result of extensive author research and review. Any recommendations for patient care must be held up against individual circumstances at hand. To the best of our knowledge any recommendations included by the author reflect currently accepted practice. However, these recommendations cannot be considered universal and complete. The authors, editor and publisher are not responsible for errors, omissions, or for any outcomes related to the use of the contents of this publication and take no responsibility for the use of the products or procedures described. Professionals using this publication should research other original sources of authority as well.

For information on this book and other continuing education materials from **PHC Publishing Group** or **PESI HealthCare**
please call **800-843-7763**
or visit our websites
www.phcpublishing.com
www.pesihealthcare.com

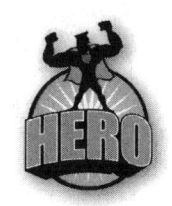

www.mobilehero.org

PHC PUBLISHING GROUP

PHC Publishing Group is an imprint of:

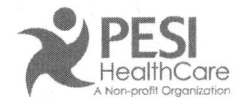

PESI HealthCare
A Non-profit Organization

Continuing Education Provider since 1979

Cover Art: Heidi Knower

Foreword

Over the last few years, we have all become familiar with the epidemic of obesity, not only the amount, but of more concern, the increase in obesity amongst children. As a mother of two, and an educator in health, fitness and nutrition, it is ingrained in me to help people strive towards wellness, by making them aware of how we can take responsibility and provide knowledge to help our children to grow into healthy adults. My older child is a nursing student and I feel that this book would be an excellent resource for her as she finds her role in any scenario of healthcare or in any healthcare setting. I have known Debbie for many years, and she has played many roles in my life. She has been my indoor cycling instructor, and motivated me to keep pursuing classes. She advised me well and was a great source of information in making the decision for my daughter to study nursing. I have always admired her dedication and passion in promoting good health across all ages and abilities. I share that passion with Debbie, along with understanding the importance of making available good, reliable, credible information that can be used by healthcare professionals to help curb childhood obesity. Her partnership with Sherrin only adds to the creativity and credibility of the book and its concepts. Sherrin is an amazing example of dedication and focus in stressing the importance of nutrition and physical activity in health promotion and health education

The HERO Guide to Health is a great resource directed to the nursing professional, but has words of wisdom for everyone and anyone interested in curbing the obesity epidemic. This makes it unique. The book may not solve the problem, but it certainly creates awareness, and will give the reader the tools to help understand, assess, and implement strategies to help fight the obesity epidemic, through health education and promotion.

I am honored to have been asked to write this foreword. This book can be used as an instructional manual to help the reader, be it a medical professional, or simply a parent who wants their child to live a healthy life. As adults, we can all use this material also, making us role models for our children. As a mother of two, a mother of a future nurse, and an educator and promoter of health and health education, I believe this book will guide you through, step by step, how to begin building a better life for you, and those around you.

Dr. Shahla Khan, PhD
University of North Florida
Brooks College of Health
Jacksonville, Florida

Preface

Obesity has become a national concern, affecting over 73 million adults, and 12 million children and adolescents (Institute of Medicine, 2012). Even a decade ago, in 2000, poor nutrition and physical inactivity were the second and third leading causes of preventable death in children, and were considered the leading causes of the obesity epidemic (Mokdad et. al, 2000). These obesity trends are rising, not falling, and leading to increased health disparities by race and ethnicity, even among children and adolescents (Ogden & Carroll, 2010). Obesity statistics are undeniable, and have been researched across many health-related fields (medicine, nursing, nutrition, psychology, behavioral health, etc…); there remains a challenge of how to reduce obesity through effective health education and intervention.

The United States of America (U.S.) obesity epidemic now affects the long-term physical, emotional, and socio-economic welfare of individuals, families, communities, and society at large. More and more children and adults are struggling with obesity-related chronic illnesses including diabetes, hypertension, heart disease, cancer, joint conditions, and more. Obesity prevention and appropriate intervention are crucial components to reverse the trend, but how can this be done? Nurses must acquire the skills to cope and intervene with this epidemic as it permeates all races, cultures, and socioeconomic groups across the United States.

<u>The HERO Guide to Health</u> will explain the vital role of the nurse in implementing multidisciplinary and collaborative strategies to assess, diagnose, implement, and increase health promotion to reduce obesity among patients and families. With over 3 million nurses in the health care workforce, nurses must become leaders, innovators, and educators in the field of health promotion and health education (Institute of Medicine, 2010). Since the time of Florence Nightingale, the role of nurse has clearly transformed, yet the role of a nurse as health promoter and patient advocate must continue to evolve. Armed with evidence-based knowledge, critical thinking skills, and cultural sensitivity, nurses will learn how to advocate for and empower their patients to make the best health choices possible.

Preface

Using the commonly used SOAP (Subjective, Objective, Assessment, Plan) format, this guide is categorized into four parts. A brief summary of the layout is as follows:

Part I: Subjective
- What is Obesity?
- Obesity & Determinants of Health
- Health & Food Culture Around the World

Part II: Objective
- Health History, Review of Systems & Obesity
- Obesity, Clinical Findings & Physical Examination
- Underlying Disability & Obesity

Part III: Assessment
- Know Your Patient: Health Assessment
- Adolescence, Health & Obesity
- Adult Health & Obesity
- Maternal Health & Obesity
- Obesity & Older Adults

Part IV: Plan
- Nutrition & Obesity in Daily Life
- Fitness Plans: When, How & Why
- Health Advocacy: How to Be Your Own HERO©

Just as nurses are accustomed to developing, implementing, and evaluating a plan set forth by a nursing or medical diagnosis, this guide will help you understand how the *prevention of obesity* or the *diagnosis of obesity* (whether formal or informal) also require goal-oriented assessments and plans to successfully care for and promote optimal health of the patient.

Throughout this guide, the authors hope to instill holistic knowledge to teach the following main objectives.

Learning Objectives:
1. Examine health assessment and physical exam in the context of obesity and health
2. Outline the elements of health that affect obesity: culture, nutrition, & fitness
3. Estimate the long-term social and physical implication of obesity
4. Describe leadership and nursing strategies to improve health promotion
5. Assess strategies for goal-setting: nutrition and fitness plans

The HERO Guide to Health is designed for the nurse and nursing professional working in a variety of healthcare and health education settings. The term "nurse" may be used to describe a nursing student, nursing assistant, licensed practical nurse, registered nurse, nurse educator, nurse practitioner, and more. Depending upon one's specific role and healthcare setting, the nurse's scope may enable more or less opportunity for educating and intervening. However, continued education for the nurse regarding the evolving healthcare needs of the community is critical for effective care in any setting.

The focus of this book is to provide a well-rounded knowledge of obesity prevention and health promotion for nursing professionals, to help promote healthy lifestyles of their clients and families. Throughout the book, we emphasize nutritional pearls for the particular age and stage of growth, we highlight the evidence-based practice to dispel misconceptions, and we provide anecdotal stories to encourage healthy habits and reduce obesity. This guide not only includes the complex nuances of physical exams among obese patients, it also provides a background to understand basic nutrition and wellness for all. This guide is not intended to replace referrals to specialists, and nurses are encouraged to make the necessary referrals for further workups and medical concerns.

References

Institute of Medicine (2012). Accelerating Progress in Obesity Prevention: Solving the Weight of the Nation. Glickman, D., Parker, L., Sim, L. J., Del Valle Cook, H., and Miller, EA Editors; Committee on Accelerating Progress in Obesity Prevention; Food and Nutrition Board; Retrieved on 05/15/12 at http://download.nap.edu/cart/download.cgi?&record_id=13275&free=1

Institute of Medicine (2010). The Future of Nursing: Focus on Education. Retrieved on 05/14/12 from http://www.iom.edu/~/media/Files/Report%20Files/2010/The-Future-of-Nursing/Nursing%20Education%202010%20Brief.pdf

Mokdad, A.H., Marks, J.S., Stroup, D.F., Gerberding, J.L. (2000). Actual causes of death in the United States, 2000. Journal of the American Medical Association. 291(10):1238-45.

Ogden, C. & Carroll, M. (2010). Prevalence of Obesity Among Children and Adolescents: United States, Trends 1963-1965 Through 2007-2008. National Centers for Health Statistics: retrieved on 05/15/12 at http://www.cdc.gov/obesity/childhood/data.html

Acknowledgments

In the first instance, we would like to thank Mayport Elementary School for inviting our (then new and untested) program, HERO, to your school with open arms. You welcomed us when we were just at the inception of our program, allowing us to develop strategies and best practices to ensure your students received a comprehensive program. We have loved every session with your kindergarten and first graders, and look forward to more years of participation in your wonderful school! Thank you to Yvonne Fergoson (Principal) and all the wonderful teachers and staff.

Thank you to the Board of HERO for their time, commitment, and dedication to our cause! Phil Greer, Casey Bulgin, and Wilton Blake – from our initial concept, continued fundraising ideas and grant applications, your commitment has been invaluable and so appreciated. To Eric, the Manager of Atlantic Beach Winn Dixie, your contributions of healthy food and consistent support of our program makes us understand the importance of local partnerships. And to the Winston Family YMCA for your support of our mobile program and parking space!

A special thank you to Dr. Julie Fairman of the University of Pennsylvania School of Nursing for providing a first read and valuable insights. Thank you to Dr. Lynn Wadelton for her unwavering support.

(Continued)

Acknowledgments

From Debbie: I want to thank my parents, Harold and Judy Liebowitz, and sisters Esther, Naomi, and Dina, for providing the love and emotional support during my youth and still today. They gave me the internal strength and courage to tackle any of life's big struggles and joys. And certainly, my children, Elliot (9) and Abby (12), have been a continued inspiration to me. I love you! They have taken our HERO cause to heart and have helped create newsletters and even short movies to support our cause! To Sherrin, I certainly could not have, and would not have, done all this without you!

From Sherrin: I'd like to thank my parents (all the way in Australia), Cheryl Whiteman and Bob Hiles, who have been and continue to be there for me in every capacity. Thanks to my Dad, Dean Whiteman, for the autonomy to live my life and follow my aspirations. To Debbie – it's the end of one journey and the beginning of another for us.

From both of us: Thank you to the team at PHC Publishing Group / PESI HealthCare, most notably Heidi Strosahl Knower for encouraging our idea and sticking with us during the entire process. Your support has been invaluable. To our preliminary editor, Barb Caffrey, your ideas added more depth and perspective to our final product and we are truly grateful.

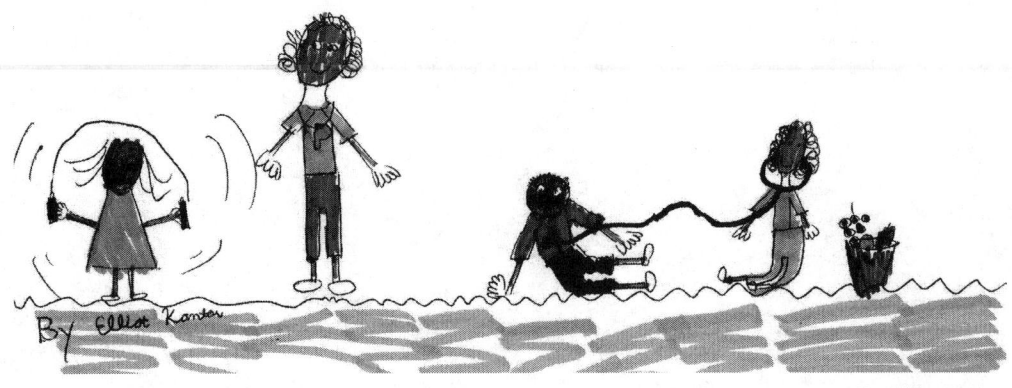

By Elliot Kantor

TABLE OF CONTENTS

Foreword iii
Preface v
Acknowledgments ix
Authors' Letters of Inclusion xii

Introduction Who Are We? ...Why We Need Obesity Prevention Programs 1

Part I: Subjective   5

Chapter 1   What is Obesity? 7
Chapter 2   Obesity & Determinants of Health 19
Chapter 3   Health & Food Culture Around the World 33

Part II: Objective   53

Chapter 4   Health History, Review of Systems & Obesity 55
Chapter 5   Obesity, Clinical Findings & Physical Examination 65
Chapter 6   Underlying Disability & Obesity 79

Part III: Assessment   95

Chapter 7   Know Your Patient: Health Assessment 97
Chapter 8   Adolescence, Health & Obesity 117
Chapter 9   Adult Health & Obesity 133
Chapter 10 Maternal Health & Obesity 147
Chapter 11 Obesity & Older Adults 157

Part IV: Plan   169

Chapter 12 Nutrition & Obesity in Daily Life 171
Chapter 13 Fitness Plans: When, How & Why 181
Chapter 14 Health Advocacy: How to Be Your Own HERO© 197

Appendices

Appendix A: SOAP Notes 207
Appendix B: Obesity 101 209
Appendix C: HERO Recipe for Success 211
Appendix D: HERO Fitness Plan 217
Appendix E: HERO Menu 219
Appendix F: Sleep Diary 221
Appendix G: Resources & Referrals 223

Authors' Letters of Inclusion

Many of us have our own stories to share. Some of us, perhaps, were not the overweight ones directly, but as nurses we have all encountered a story that somehow affects us.

We share with you our own stories to highlight how our personal experiences have contributed to the work we do today. Nurses do not always have the firsthand experience to know the physical and emotional toll an illness takes on the patient, but having experienced something similar, one can better relate, comprehend, and feel compassion for the individual.

As you read these two stories, consider this:

- How are the personal stories similar? And how are they different?
- What could have improved our experiences? Medically? Socially?
- What would be the health concerns for each story?

Debbie's Story

I was an "overweight" child from age 7 until age 15, during the formative years. During the earlier years, I do not recall "feeling fat," but by age ten, I certainly felt different from the rest of the kids. And by junior high, I definitely knew I was larger than most kids my age. Calculating my BMI based on my measurements then, by today's calculations, I was obese with a BMI near 30. At that time, I considered myself overweight, not obese. Though chubby, pudgy, plump would have been coined for me too. I knew I didn't like my size.

At 5'2" and weighing over 160 pounds, I was not just "big-boned" or "short for my weight." I was obese at a time when most children were not. While I did not have diabetes, I did (and still do) have asthma. I attributed my difficulty in gym class to my asthma, though clearly my added weight added greater challenge too. Either way, I needed P.E. more than anyone, yet found the class embarrassing since I just could not keep up.

I was the chubby kid who, friendly but shy, was insecure; I was sure that people were whispering about *me* whenever I saw people congregate nearby. And, unfortunately, sometimes they were. I still had friends, and didn't let my size fully take over my spirit, though I did feel a damper on spirit and confidence.

In 1985, I had the added challenge of spending the year abroad in the Middle East, with my family. I had left my American friends for a year in Israel. A new culture, new language, new foods, and hopefully new friends. Luckily, I met a few Americans and at least had less of a language barrier than expected, but I still stuck out as not only the American with poor language skills, but also the heavy child. I made friends, but also was teased by some children. My appearance as a short-haired chubby kid in a all-girl class, I suppose, gave the illusion of me as a tough girl. Yet, I was tormented and teased, and children physically gave me what we then called "Indian burns" by twisting my arm. I was laughed at in gym class when we had to dress out in tight blue polyester shorts and white T-shirt, and I still remember being pegged by a dodgeball and laughed at during a school tournament.

I had to cope with a new place, new foods, and new way of life. And it was difficult. This was Israel, in the 1980s, where people walked everywhere. Even at age six, children were walking the city streets to go buy bread and milk. Rainy winter, or muggy summer, we walked and walked. While I did need the exercise, walking in the heat of summer was the bane of my existence. At ages ten, eleven, and twelve, I was miserable walking in the sweaty heat. On the outside, I was chubby and slower than my peers, but on the inside, my legs burned as they rubbed together under my skirt. Baby powder sprinkled on my inner thighs, or shorts worn under my skirt to prevent friction rubbing, offered no reprieve from the pain of skin on skin. I remember getting home with chaffed thighs from the sweaty walk. But it was not only there, in Israel, where my added pounds took a toll on me physically and emotionally.

In America, before and after that year abroad, I played on a softball team from age 9 and had daily physical education (P.E.) at school, unlike the sparse gym classes today. I ate foods prepared at home, and lunches prepared by my loving mother. And still, I was fat. It was physically and emotionally painful. I will never forget how humiliating and embarrassing it was for me when, in my seventh grade gym class, students individually had to "weigh in" on the stage of the gymnasium while other students all sat on the gym floor waiting for their names to be called. Though the weights were not announced, students clearly were watching and asking the weights of their peers.

I have never cheated on any test before and never did again, but I cheated this time. My name was called; I walked up onto the stage and stepped onto the scale beside the coach's desk. I pressed my thumb as hard as I could onto the coach's desk and voila! I shaved off 10 pounds instantly! Brilliant and deceptive.

Did I do myself a favor? No. Did I go home and talk to my parents about needing to lose weight? I don't think so. I was young and embarrassed. Perhaps that event spared me slight humiliation by weighing 150 pounds instead of 160 pounds at age 13. I knew I was overweight and thought that embarrassment was enough.

(I share this with you to emphasize the importance of sensitivity towards children and adults alike. Even if we know we need help, privacy and senstivity should be ensured by the nurse and staff to prevent any additional embarrassment.)

It took me another two years to build the inner strength to make necessary changes, even though I was determined to lose weight. First, I tried many fad diets, losing and gaining a few pounds here and there, but that ultimately didn't help anything. So when I was fifteen, I decided to harness my inner strength and tackle a new pattern of eating and exercise. While this was partly because I didn't feel either "girly" or sexy, and partly again because I was afraid boys would never like me if I stayed the way I was, I also wanted to be more healthy for my own sake.

My new mantra was "eat to live, don't live to eat." While I have always truly loved food, I decided that eating should not be either my hobby or my favorite pastime. Instead, I decided to eat for the health of my body.

I committed to a more healthy lifestyle, and stuck with it for the next six months. During this time, I learned what was needed to maintain a healthy weight over time. I remember making myself tuna salads for lunch every day; at dinners with my family, I had a small portion of the pasta dish of the night, but otherwise fortified my plate with a variety of protein and calcium-rich foods, salads and whole grains. I made sure that every meal consisted of multiple types of foods so I felt that I was eating more.

All of this helped me to approach food from a different perspective. I realized that my downfall was eating salty snacks like potato chips, as I could easily devour a large bagful in one sitting. The sodium, the fat, and the carbohydrates in that bag of chips were the main contributors to my obesity.

For exercise, I began riding a stationary bicycle that had previously sat, unused, with laundry piling up on it, in my parents' room. Right around the debut of Jonny G's Spinning fad, but without my knowledge of it, and without a gym membership, I began indoor cycling. While I studied for my freshman biology tests or while watching television, my legs were spinning.

Weight loss was slow but steady. And I stuck with it! How did I do it? Slow and steady. Had I given up within even two months, I would have seen little to no results. (Remember that my goal was weight loss, though for others, the goal is overall health without actually losing weight). Fifteen years later, I became a spinning instructor.

To succeed with my goal of weight loss I followed these personal priorities:

- 50% *patience* (do *not* give up)
- 30% focus on eating fewer calories (but nutritionally dense calories)
- 20% focus on exercising more (cardiovascular exercise)

By tenth grade, I had lost 44 pounds and felt fresh and new! For the first time, boys started to notice me and I had my first boyfriend. I enjoyed clothing shopping, and wore a bathing suit without wearing a T-shirt cover-up and shorts to hide my body. I began tucking shirts in to show off my new waistline.

But inside, there was something upsetting. With the new me, I realized how people *do* judge and stigmatize overweight people. This was extremely distressing. I had been fat and I struggled with it for many years, but most people didn't see me for who I was – they just saw my weight and external appearance. I knew that was the case when people *did* treat me differently when I was overweight – and when I was not.

That's what caused me to realize that society is quick to place blame on the individual without regard to the food, culture, and environment that influences us. This made me ponder a few things over the next few decades. Does and *should* America blame the American culture of fast food and urban sprawl, or does and *should* society shift blame to the individual? Is obesity caused by sheer overeating, denial, cultural patterns, or lack of health education or self-advocacy?

Sherrin's Story

I grew up and have spent most of my life in Australia, which has a different culture, different foods and a very different lifestyle than is typically seen in the United States. I was always a tall, skinny child; through adolescence my weight remained steady. By the time I was seventeen, I was 5'10" and weighed 140 pounds.

My weight was never an issue for me growing up. I played sports during school hours, took basketball or some type of sport three afternoons a week, and went to the gym four afternoons a week, as I enjoyed exercising. Because of this, and because I came from a home with a diet heavy in salads and grilled meat, I never really had to think about what I was eating.

At seventeen, I joined the Royal Australian Navy, and entered the Naval Academy where, over four years, I would earn my degree as well as learn the required military specialist skills. Having been very active throughout my life, the fitness components were not difficult, and at first, I enjoyed the new lifestyle that I had merged into.

But there was a looming problem. For the first time, I could eat and drink what I liked, with all main meals served in a cafeteria-style setting. Three meals a day, seven days a week, there were hot, calorie-laden meals available. Additionally, once I turned eighteen, I was able to legally drink alcohol (as the legal drinking age in Australia is eighteen). Therefore, I began to steadily drink beer and eat pizza with the rest of my colleagues.

In a six month period, I managed to gain almost 40 pounds and, while I recognized the weight gain, most of my counterparts had also gained weight, so I assumed I could lose it just as easily as I had gained it. As I'm quite tall at 5'10", I could "hide" some of the weight and people would always comment, "It's okay; you are tall."

I knew that I had to lose weight, but over the course of the next ten years, my weight would spiral up and down dramatically. While I was at the Academy, I lost 25 pounds very quickly through a terrible diet of eating only vegetables and two glasses of milk with a piece of fruit a day. While the weight came off, I was slower, had no energy and found it difficult to maintain the standard level of fitness.

After I lost weight, the diet I had was not sustainable. I soon resumed my old eating habits and, without noticing, I quickly put the 25 pounds back on.

What I couldn't understand (and what frustrated me) was that I was always active. While my levels of physical activity were less than they were in high school, I was still partaking in regular physical activity, and I didn't think my eating was that bad. (In hindsight, I understand now that my portions were too big and I was eating the wrong foods).

I continually tried different diets, not eating, over-exercising; I really couldn't stick to one thing. If I didn't see results in three or four days, I would get depressed and the cycle would start again.

Being in a male-dominated military environment, it was difficult for me to have the extra weight, not only because I felt slower and unattractive, but because I thought people were judging me. Even though I was bigger, I was still fit and very strong. But because I was overweight, I felt disgusting and really didn't want to be around anyone.

The military is a unique environment. I didn't want to show weakness and, because I am a public speaker, I know how to exude confidence on the outside. No one really knew how I felt internally, which I'd now characterize as 'exceptionally depressed."

I arrived in the USA in November of 2008. I knew that I wasn't content. I had a great job, a fantastic apartment, a brand new car and a new life to start, but at 180 pounds, I wasn't happy with myself. I met new people, all of whom were thin and attractive, and although they were very friendly, I always felt out of place.

America is an entirely different country than Australia. Here in the U.S., I was bombarded with television and radio commercials offering quick and easy fixes for weight loss and, at one stage, I was convinced to try liposuction. However, I thought better of it and never went.

February of 2009 was when I decided to lose weight. I vowed to myself that I would do it, but I never told anyone for fear of not reaching a goal or seeing any results. So I kept it to myself and came up with my own eating and workout plan.

The first month was terrible. I saw no results and was upset, feeling as though I was a failure. But I decided to persevere, because I was sick of looking like I did. The eating plan I devised involved eating regularly, making better food choices, and not eating because others were or because I felt like I should. Instead, I ate when I was hungry and reduced my alcohol consumption. I didn't remove anything from my diet; instead, I changed portions and made better choices.

But it wasn't easy. It took hard work and perseverance to change my habits and lifestyle. I worked out every day and made the time. I would work out at lunch, after work, or even before work (which I really don't enjoy to this day). Working out soon became a habit, one that I knew was going to help me eventually.

After five months, my parents visited (in June; they had not seen me since November, 2008). They saw that I had lost weight (as I now weighed 165 pounds). Their comments that I looked better and healthier were really a boost. Friends had also noticed and commented; although I felt better, I wasn't done.

By this point, my routine was regimented and I felt better. I still would have a few beers, but I ate lots more salads and vegetables and I was enjoying working out. My habits were now my lifestyle.

It wasn't for another year until my parents saw me again. By this point, I was 135 pounds; they were blown away. Friends whom I hadn't seen in a few months were shocked and asked me how I had done it. I told them perseverance and hard work. At a routine doctor appointment, the doctor insisted that I had taken some form of pharmaceutical to assist in the weight loss; at no stage was that true.

As of February, 2012, my weight is currently 132-135 pounds. I don't weigh myself often, but I do work out, I do eat well and I do enjoy life. I eat cheesecake (though usually half a slice), indulge in an alcoholic beverage or two, and feel great mentally and physically.

What I learned through it all is that weight loss is unique to the individual: it's difficult, it's frustrating and it's an emotional roller coaster. It's a slow, laborious process that happens over time and takes a persistent mental fortitude and a desire to change habits and transform those habits into beliefs and values

Once you see and feel the results, you never want to go back. I feel emancipated to a degree, not only with the weight loss, but with the satisfaction of knowing I did it, as an individual without any potion, fad or craze.

The causes of obesity are highly complex, as personal behaviors, environmental influences, and cultural ideals are often intertwined. Our patients, like us, have very different experiences that can affect us positively and/or negatively. The challenge is to encourage patients to work towards a positive outcome by promoting health and encouraging our patients to take active steps to either reduce obesity or prevent obesity. Realizing that one's physical and social environments do impact the likelihood of becoming obese is a first step towards recognizing the positive changes we can make in our own environments.

Authors' Letters of Inclusion

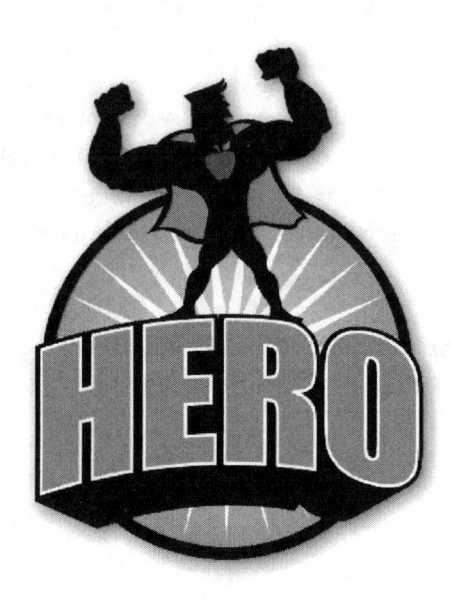

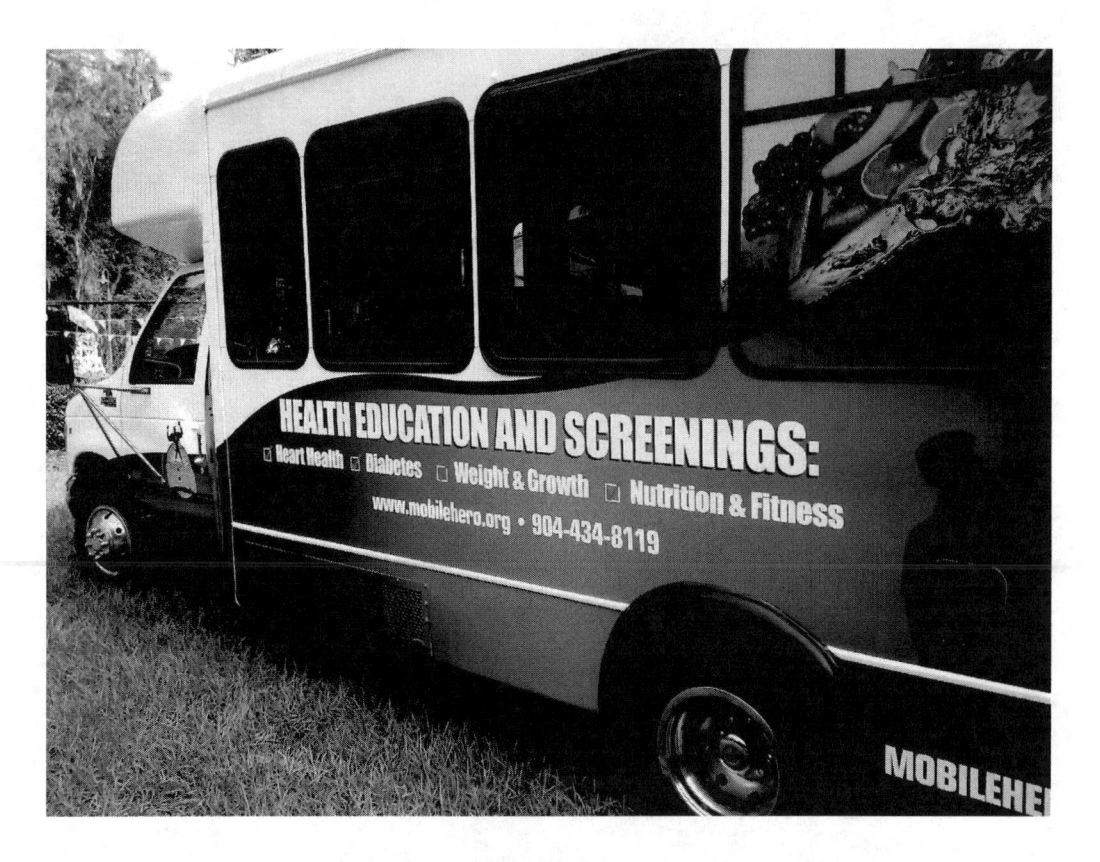

HERO Mobile Health: Our vision for obesity prevention and health promotion has come to life!

Introduction

Who Are We?
...Why We Need Obesity Prevention Programs

Childhood obesity has become a widespread and increasing public health concern, both nationally and internationally. Although obesity and weight gain can be attributed to a concept as simple as increased caloric intake and decreased energy expenditure, the complexity of variables affecting children and adults across cultures and their individual lifespans has created a dramatic public health challenge. Obesity cannot be attributed to one causative factor, as each individual's unique environment, genetic disposition, health knowledge, and other health determinants affect the likelihood of becoming obese. Not only has childhood obesity become a national health concern, but so have the direct health consequences of obesity (including heart disease and diabetes among more children and adults). All of these issues, in combination, have taken a toll physically, emotionally, and financially on the health of this country. And while the need for intervention is known, how to accomplish this remains to be determined. In this introduction, we explain how the HERO Program was initiated as a call to action to combat childhood obesity.

Just as the causes for obesity are multifactorial, so are the methods of preventing and treating it. Family-based, school-based, community-based, and healthcare-based interventions have been explored, and public health policies are now improving access and funding for such programming (Karnik & Kanekar, 2012). In an effort to both improve healthcare and reduce health-related expenditures in the United States, President Obama signed the Affordable Care Act in 2010. Under this plan, preventative medicine would now become a greater focus, both to reduce spending and to improve health via preventing illness. With $25 million allocated to creating a systematic and comprehensive model for reducing obesity, the Department of Health and Human Services began expanding campaigns to fight obesity, in hopes that each state and health department would increase preventative services (The White House, 2010). While federal funds have been allocated towards health initiatives, this occurs at a time of significant budget reforms for the educational systems. Within the school system, there is recognition of the need for health promotion, yet there is also a lack of infrastructure and budget to provide once mandatory physical education programs. Thus, despite health reforms, mandates, and certain health initiatives and programs, there remains an upward trend towards higher obesity rates and a lack of consistency across programs that should essentially interlink and compliment one another.

The founders of HERO discovered that it is not the theory of obesity prevention that must be addressed, but rather the methods of providing direct intervention. Although there are programs that target nutrition and fitness in various settings, there is a lack of comprehensive programs that directly include health education from a medical perspective in combination with nutrition and fitness education. The inception of HERO was partly formulated after the founders realized that there was a distinct gap between general health programs and direct programming to help explain WHY and HOW health is affected by nutrition and physical activity. For the HERO team, childhood obesity seemed to be a perfect focus for initiating targeted change.

HERO (Health Education to Reduce Obesity) began as a grassroots program with a mission to combat childhood obesity through hands-on health education, fitness, and nutrition programming for children. Recognizing that there is a severe gap between the health policies and the actual implementation of health education for children and families, HERO was created to fill this gap and supplement what should be provided through the Department of Health and Department of Education.

With only an initial concept of how to accomplish this, we, Debbie Kantor (a nurse practitioner) and Sherrin Whiteman (a navy lieutenant) serendipitously formulated a novel approach to the obesity epidemic. HERO evolved through the merging of two essentially different ideas. Debbie's idea was to start a food truck, which would teach families in lower socioeconomic areas about healthy cooking techniques. After hearing the idea, Sherrin was quick to respond that nutrition education is only one essential part of healthy living, and physical activity is just as imperative. So the idea evolved to teach not only nutrition and healthy cooking, but also incorporate fitness activities for these families.
With this newly-focused concept, HERO quickly started developing relations with local county schools and the Health Department through research of existing programs aimed at reducing childhood obesity. The HERO team soon recognized that, while there are many policies in place, there is a disparate amount of effective hands-on programmatic activities linking young people to needed health programs.

Armed with a goal to form a holistic, hands-on health education program, HERO took the challenge and approached Mayport Elementary in Jacksonville,

Florida. Mayport Elementary, a Title 1 school with over 70% of the students on free or reduced lunch, fell geographically within one the city's Health Zones. We explained the HERO idea to the principal, Ms. Yvonne Ferguson, and she agreed to have HERO pilot the concept with Kindergarten classes. HERO now teaches its program to all First Grade classes at the school, with teachers reporting a heightened level of nutrition and fitness education. The classes are met with exuberance from the children, who look forward to trying new foods with Debbie and running around with Sherrin.

The HERO program continues to gain momentum and, in 2012, received approval from the Duval County School Health Advisory Council (SHAC), which enables the HERO program to provide its services in Elementary Schools throughout Duval County. Already in regular attendance at Parent Teacher Events and School Open Days, HERO is collaborating with the Parent Teacher Advisory Council to provide family education classes and family activity days.

HERO is the first mobile health program led by a nurse practitioner and navy lieutenant that provides health education directly to elementary students. Participating classes receive a one-hour session every other week. Sessions are divided into two 30- minute segments. Sherrin leads one class through a fitness circuit with games, team drills and aerobic activities, while Debbie leads a 30-minute health program to educate the students about USDA food recommendations, body systems, nutrition and health. The classes then swap, so that each student receives both health and fitness sessions during the one-hour time period. The students receive 8 sessions over 16 weeks and, by the end of the program, even six year-old students can answer such questions as:

- How big is the heart?
- What is the function of the heart?
- Why do we measure blood pressure?
- What is the purpose of blood, muscles, bones, etc.?
- What are the essential food groups and why do we eat them?
- What is fiber? Protein? A calorie? Fat?
- Why and how do we monitor growth (height/weight/BMI)?
- How does fitness affect your heart?
- What activities can you do to strengthen muscles, bones, etc.?
- Why do we need to drink plenty of water?

What makes the HERO program unique is that we provide a comprehensive look at health from a medical perspective. Not only do we strive to educate people to eat healthier and exercise, we teach them WHY it is important and how, as individuals, we can make a difference in our own health. Many other

Introduction

programs look at one or two facets of healthy living, focusing either on the theories behind fitness and healthy eating, or providing demonstrative classes that lack the theory and educational prose to elicit change. HERO provides both theoretical knowledge and hands-on programmatic activities for both fitness and nutrition concurrently while supplementing current school curriculums.

As the program evolves, HERO remains a mobile multidisciplinary school and community-based project that aims to combat childhood obesity through a combination of hands-on nutrition education, fitness training and healthy lifestyle promotion. We believe that, by generating health literacy and education, we are enabling individuals to increase control over their health and risk factors, and thereby improve health-related knowledge, attitudes, motivation, confidence, behavioral intentions and personal skills concerning healthy lifestyles, as well as knowledge of how to access information and implement healthy lifestyles.

References

Karnik, S. & Kanekar, A. (2012). Childhood Obesity: A Global Public Health Crisis. International Journal of Preventative Medicine. January; 3(1): 1–7. Retrieved on 05/16/12 at http://www.ncbi.nlm.nih.gov/pmc/articles/PMC3278864/

The White House. Health Reform for Children: The Affordable Care Act Gives Parents Greater Control Over Their Children's Health Care http://www.whitehouse.gov/files/documents/health_reform_for_children.pdf

PART I: SUBJECTIVE

In Part I, we explore individual, environmental, cultural, and public health issues as they relate to the obesity epidemic. Obesity must be understood not only clinically, but holistically and subjectively, and across all ages and populations. For nurses to tackle the nuances of patient care related to obesity and wellness, they must first understand the sociological context of the individual, and the interplay between the patient and nurse in the community and society as a whole. Within Chapters 1, 2, & 3, we examine the subjective meaning of obesity, various health determinants, and health culture across the globe. Nurses and our patients must identify obesity as a problem before we can examine, assess and plan effective strategies to reduce obesity and/or promote health for individuals, communities, and society at large. The role of the nurse is crucial to first identifying obesity or the risk of obesity among patients and communities.

Chapter 1
What is Obesity?

To understand the meaning of obesity, The HERO Guide to Health, explores not only obesity per se, but also related health conditions, and cultural and environmental differences that affect nutrition, fitness, and overall health. Primary prevention to reduce obesity will remain a theme throughout this guide. Our special interest in childhood obesity (per the introduction) highlights the need for early intervention and education, though it must be understood that prevention can also be successful later in life among those already overweight, obese, and/or and chronically ill.

Part I will help to explain why and how health culture and perceptions can increase obesity, and increase the risk of other health conditions such as diabetes and heart disease. While many people equate being "thin" with being "healthy," and being overweight or obese with being "unhealthy," neither assumption is necessarily true. Thus, this guide is intended to promote health for all patients of any weight or health status. Nurses will learn how changes in nutrition and health habits have led to increased obesity and a significant public health concern.

> Chapter 1 Objectives:
> 1. Discuss the rising obesity trends among children and adults
> 2. Identify obesity as a public health problem
> 3. Estimate the social impact of obesity
> 4. Summarize the role of the nurse

Obesity Trends

Childhood obesity has more than quadrupled among 6- to 11-year-olds, and tripled among 12- to 19-year-olds over the past three decades, and related chronic illnesses including diabetes, heart disease, and hypertension are on the rise (Active Living Research, 2011). It is estimated that over 23 million young adults are overweight or obese in this country. No doubt obesity has become a major health crisis in this country for the young and adult populations. Federal programs and lawmakers, hospitals and health providers, communities and organizations are searching and researching ways to improve the health of our population and individuals. Left untreated and without effective intervention, the Institute of Medicine (2012) predicts that obesity and related conditions will cause a decline in health, obesity-related healthcare costs that exceed 190 billion dollars, and catastrophic repercussions for our workforce and general population. The Institute of Medicine found that two thirds of adults and one third of children are either overweight or obese (2012).

The effects of obesity on the rates of diabetes are considerable, and The International Diabetes Federation predicts that, by 2030, *one in ten adults will have diabetes* – a staggering statistic that far exceeds that of the Centers for Disease Control in its prediction from 2001 (Diabetes Care, 2011). The significant difference is partly attributed to the number of adults living with undiagnosed diabetes. The concept that obesity increases the risk of diabetes remains relatively new and, thus, many overweight people have not recognized the need to prevent or seek medical care for diabetes or pre-diabetes.

Pharmaceutical companies are constantly improving medical treatment for diabetes, while more and more patients are diagnosed and are seeking treatment. Here lies the paradox: advanced medicine identifies what makes us healthy, and yet advanced culture more readily provides that which does not. But no single cause for this obesity epidemic takes the blame, nor is there one single cure for it. Obesity prevention and health promotion will require a multitiered intervention than incorporates not only the individual, but also the families and communities. Society must recognize this: obesity has created a complex public health problem that will require multidisciplinary and consistent interventions.

Almost daily, new statistics are disseminated and evidence shows the significant rise in obesity in this country. Even lay observers can recognize that the average size of people in America has drastically changed over the last decade. Out in public, perhaps within the confines of our own home, and in the community, we can witness what appears to be a change (over the past few decades) in average body and retail clothing sizes, average restaurant portion sizes, and the average number of readily available prepackaged foods and restaurant chains. The media, be it radio, computer-based, or television, has a preponderance of advertisements for fast food restaurants, but also bombards the public with ads for weight loss, health, and fitness centers. Subjectively, our society is changing, and so is the general health and welfare of our patients.

Despite realizing a change in general body size, many of our patients still do not know what obesity means to them or to our society. This guide will walk you through to an understanding why nurses are the key healthcare providers to tackle the obesity issue.

Obesity & Public Health

Sometimes, despite an *apparent* public health issue, legislation, litigation, and high-profile attention is needed before an issue becomes pressing enough to garner support (Mello et al., 2006). Nurses must recognize how health policy functions to improve the health of our individual patients. While this process seems tedious and inefficient at times, we must understand how health policies are an attempt to improve the public health for future generations. Historically, state governments have exercised police power (within the Tenth Amendment of the Constitution) to enforce or regulate the private sector for the welfare of the public. Such legislation can include enforcing taxation on food items or providing warnings or placing limits on advertising (as in the case of tobacco use in America).

As early as 2000, 19 states already enforced some food taxation of sugared beverages and snack foods (Mello et al., 2006). There is a wide variation in intervention and active reform, though momentum is gaining to increase awareness of the needs of the public. Policital figures and their causes, like Michelle Obama and her "Let's Move Campaign" and former President Bill Clinton and his "Alliance for a Healthier Generation," have become well renowned for their advocacy in the field of obesity. And lesser known programs have begun to sprout up, like our own HERO program. This continued public health awareness by groups both large and small can eventually lead to sound intervention that can help reduce the rates of obesity over time.

But, until then, the fight against the obesity epidemic, now reminiscent of the challenge of reducing smoking and cigarette use among young and old alike, will require public health initiatives together with action at a more tangible level (strategies that you as nurse can provide directly). In 2001, the Surgeon General's report on obesity helped gain recognition for the need for health reforms related to obesity, yet, unfortunately, with awareness sometimes comes criticism and fear of impinging on civil liberties. And thus, another paradox ensues: people want the right to sue for damages, yet the right to purchase that which may be deleterious to them.

The notorious lawsuit against McDonald's® waxed and waned for several years, and spurred considerable media attention, including films like "Super Size Me" that demonstrated how eating fast food consistently can affect one's health even over a short time. As always, there remains the challenge of exercising individual versus government control and responsibility. Most recently, Mayor Bloomberg of New York has proposed a ban on sugared beverages, in an attempt to reduce the primary source of added calories, which contributes to the obesity epidemic. By the time this book is printed, we shall see a decision regarding this proposal, which would give restaurants and vendors nine months to conform, or

1: What is Obesity?

face fees and penalties, as a way to discourage the sale of soft drinks. Is this the solution? We think not. This is a mere "tip of the iceberg" and certainly does not solve a complex problem in a comprehensive manner.

Despite this age-old dilemma (and conflicting messages by the media, lobbyists, corporations, and individuals), federal programs remain responsible for regulating certain practices. With the obesity crisis, federal programs are stepping up efforts to improve food- and health-related services. In the nutrition and food sector, the Food and Drug Administration (FDA) has been regulating food nutrition labels since 1994, and continues to promote food safety, and increase awareness of nutritional needs (as we will see in the coming chapters). Similarly, Medicare followed healthcare reform by newly defining obesity as a medical disease (HHS, 2004), and thus has created awareness and support for fitness, nutrition, and obesity counseling. Steadily, more programs and initiatives are addressing childhood obesity and increased rates of diabetes and heart disease, and helping to raise awareness of the effect of these conditions on individual health.

Clearly, federal and public health initiatives are necessary, and certainly they can fill some of the gaps for under insured and disabled individuals. But, how can we help our patients to understand the importance of individual health and how it affects public health and vice versa? Nurses must help patients understand that ,while the individual is at the core, there are influencing powers that surround us: our environment, government, and community. Helping patients understand how to become empowered through using health resources within these surrounding elements can improve not only the individual's health, but also that of the public over time.

In the context of obesity, our patients must understand the role of *individual* responsibility regarding healthy choices. That is, given what is available, what are the best choices regarding foods they eat, activities, and elimination of habits that are health risks (like smoking, drinking, etc?) The surrounding influences should be identified as *resources* to help contribute to better health. The nurse can help patients identify harmful influences as well as those which are healthful, such as:

1. Community resources: charitable organizations, food pantries, YMCA, support programs, etc.
2. Federal programs: how to access Medicaid, Medicare, Social Security,etc.
3. Family and environmental resources: how to make use of parks and family time
4. Work-related resources: gym or stairs at work, food choices at work, etc.
5. Medical resources: clinics that may offer free screenings or health information

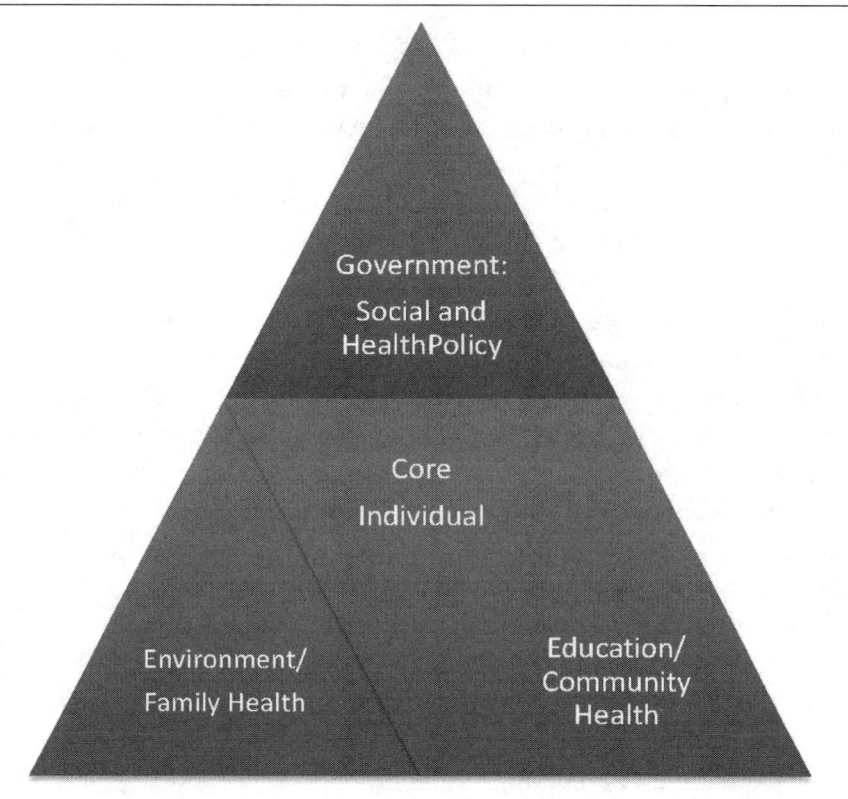

```
                    Government:
                    Social and
                    HealthPolicy


                      Core
                    Individual


        Environment/              Education/
        Family Health             Community
                                    Health
```

© 2012 HERO Inc.

Figure 1-1. Your Patient as the Core Individual

As a health activists (as we all are in some ways – whether actively or by default – as nurses and healthcare providers), nurses must work in unison to foster health promotion and obesity prevention measures. Helping your patients understand how the health education that you provide them is tailored to fit their unique situations can help empower them to make self-motivated choices.

The Social Impact of Obesity

We recognize that the word "obesity" means different things to different people. It is a word that is often seen as stigmatizing, as it has significant negative connotations, especially among non-medical people. As nurses, we know that obesity has its *clinical* definition (calculated ratios of body measurements) and a *lay* definition, meaning a largely overweight person. Nurses must understand the interplay between both the medical and social aspects of obesity.

As we will examine in Part II, clinical obesity is a more concrete definition and measurement and thus, perhaps easier for the patient to understand. But, obesity needs to be defined *not* just as a measurement of height, weight, and BMI, or even just in the context of the physical exam. We will explain the

I: What is Obesity?

process of taking a health history and review of systems related to obesity, and will also learn to take a physical exam in PART III. But for now, we address obesity as a subjective yet ubiquitous term.

Obesity is not a topic most of us have studied rigorously, nor are we as nurses prepared for the consequences of caring for obese children and adults. In nursing school, we learn and teach physical exam of the healthy patient, to help identify what is atypical for that person. But, we do know that obesity is a consequence of a long-standing pattern; in other words, people become overweight or obese *over time*. (Note that a sudden weight gain should certainly be explored as there may acute reasons for this, such as fluid retention from heart failure, liver disease, thyroid conditions, etc.) Generally, weight gain is a progression and is not sudden or acute. And obesity, without prevention or intervention, can be a lifelong battle. So how do we assess what seems to be general and non-clinical? And how do we introduce the subjectivity of obesity into the clinical setting?

As nurses, we are likely the **first pass** for the patient before he/she reaches the stage of diagnosis. Recognizing *subjectively* what obesity means within the patient's frame of mind is crucial. If we do not make a point of assessing what is seemingly obvious, as a nursing problem, then it will likely be ignored once the patient is deeper in the medical arena of visits for other clinical conditions. When we care for a patient who is overweight, obese, or at risk, they likely come to us with some already preconceived notion of what obesity means to them in their culture, family or environment.

Understanding not only the patient's baseline health, but also their perception of health will be a highly critical portion of the health assessment. Because the perception of health may be so variable across cultures and lifestyles, that nurses must assess the health environment in all its complexities. A parent caring for an obese child will likely not seek help for the child if they do not perceive there is a problem or health risk. Remember that, even a few decades ago, being overweight or obese was not inherently "bad" for your health. In fact, culturally, some people may consider the large figure as a sign of wealth or prosperity, especially if they have experienced a lack of food resources. (Think back to Renaissance art with plump women, whose naked figures were deemed beautiful and richly painted.) In contrast, the Barbie Doll figure should not be strived for either, and nurses must understand what the patient perceives as a healthy and beautiful body type.

Obesity must be understood in the context of the patient and his or her overall health. Some patients already know they are overweight, or recognize that their children are overweight, but will not seek help because they do not understand the effect of obesity on their overall health. In our experience with

HERO, we worked with a seven-year-old African-American girl in first grade in public school in Florida. She clearly is obese, weighing 101 pounds, and is having difficulty keeping up physically with her peers. Worse yet, she already demonstrates early signs of prediabetes as, by teacher report, she drinks water excessively and urinates frequently. Teachers have spoken with her parents and they refuse to take her to the doctor. We look at research on health perception to show that, culturally, many people do not perceive obesity as a health risk and thus may not feel the need to seek medical care.

A study by Young-Hyman et al. (2000) entitled, "Care Giver Perception of Children's Obesity-Related Health Risk: A Study of African American Families," demonstrated that, although 57% and 12% of children in this study were obese or super obese (respectively), only 44% of the children's caregivers believed the children to be at a health risk. This is concerning. Similarly, research on preschool children and parental perception of obesity indicated that less than 6% of parents considered their children to have high body weight, though clinically, one third were obese or at risk of obesity (Garrett-Wright, 2011). Health literacy of the parents contributed to their ability to perceive their children as overweight or at risk, despite apparent concern for their children. This highlights the need for health education early, not only for the sake of the child, but to promote healthy habits within the home from a young age.

Public health officials have compared the obesity epidemic to smoking, which required decades of time and lawsuits to finally lead to policy change. As with smoking or any risky behavior, there must be targeted health educational interventions to help people understand *how* and *why* being or becoming overweight and obese is a clear health risk – only then can strategies be introduced to make healthy changes.

How can we emphasize the significance of obesity when it has been a social issue for so long? While there are common themes of living without disease, there are many people who consider themselves "healthy" despite their true medical condition. Ask one person what "being healthy" means, and they might say, "Being able to run a marathon." Ask another, and they might say, "Living long enough to see my grandchildren."

In Chapter 2, we will examine the determinants of health and, in Chapter 3, we will look at the health culture across the globe. But certainly we must also understand some very basic values of health and how they translate into the patient's view of obesity. Remember these questions as we proceed through the following chapters, and during conversations with your patients.

I: What is Obesity?

How Does Your Patient Value Health?

1. Is living a long life the symbol of health?
   If so, is the patient aware that obesity can reduce one's life span related to chronic disease associated with obesity (diabetes, heart disease, cancer and more)?

2. Is living free of illness, even if for a short time, the symbol of health?
   If so, is the patient aware that obese individuals have higher risk of living with one or more chronic illnesses?

3. Is having a medical condition, but overcoming it, the symbol of health?
   If so, is the patient willing and able to lose weight and reduce their risk of obesity-related health complications? This would be a promising view of health, as this view would encourage health promotion and healthful changes.

Subjectively, our patients know certain basic elements of health – what are these?

1. "Eat Well"
2. "Exercise"
3. "Don't smoke"
4. "Don't drink"
5. Maslow's Hierarchy of Needs might guide people to know the need for food, shelter, air, love, and self-actualization

The Role of the Nurse

As nurses, we must understand our own roles in the obesity epidemic, whether or not your specific job description incudes health education. The role of the nurse is to educate, promote and foster health values that are appropriate for the patient. According to the World Health Organization, the definition of a nurse is the following:

> Nursing encompasses autonomous and collaborative care of individuals of all ages, families, groups and communities, sick or well and in all settings. It includes the promotion of health, the prevention of illness, and the care of ill, disabled and dying people.
>
> (World Health Organization, 2012)

Globally, WHO recognizes that nurses make up the largest segment of the healthcare population (with an estimated 2.9 million nurses in the United States), and that their expertise is critical to public health. In 2011, the Sixty-fourth World Health Assembly focused on nurse recruitment and retention and, on recognizing the need to increase nurse education to improve health systems (WHO, 2011). WHO encouraged its members worldwide to increase collaboration with nurses to create action plans to improve patient-centered and community health. Healthcare systems and nurses alike must recognize the importance of nurses in healthcare and public health. In the context of obesity and health promotion, nurses have the ability to wear many hats, have exposure to and influence over many populations across many settings, and actively partake in and implement needed healthcare solutions. Unlike during the time of Florence Nightingale, nurses today are not just at the bedside opening windows, holding hands, and cleaning chamber pots. While there is certainly value to historical nursing, the evolution of nursing has contributed to the need for more research, evidence-based techniques, and leadership roles among nurses in the public health sector.

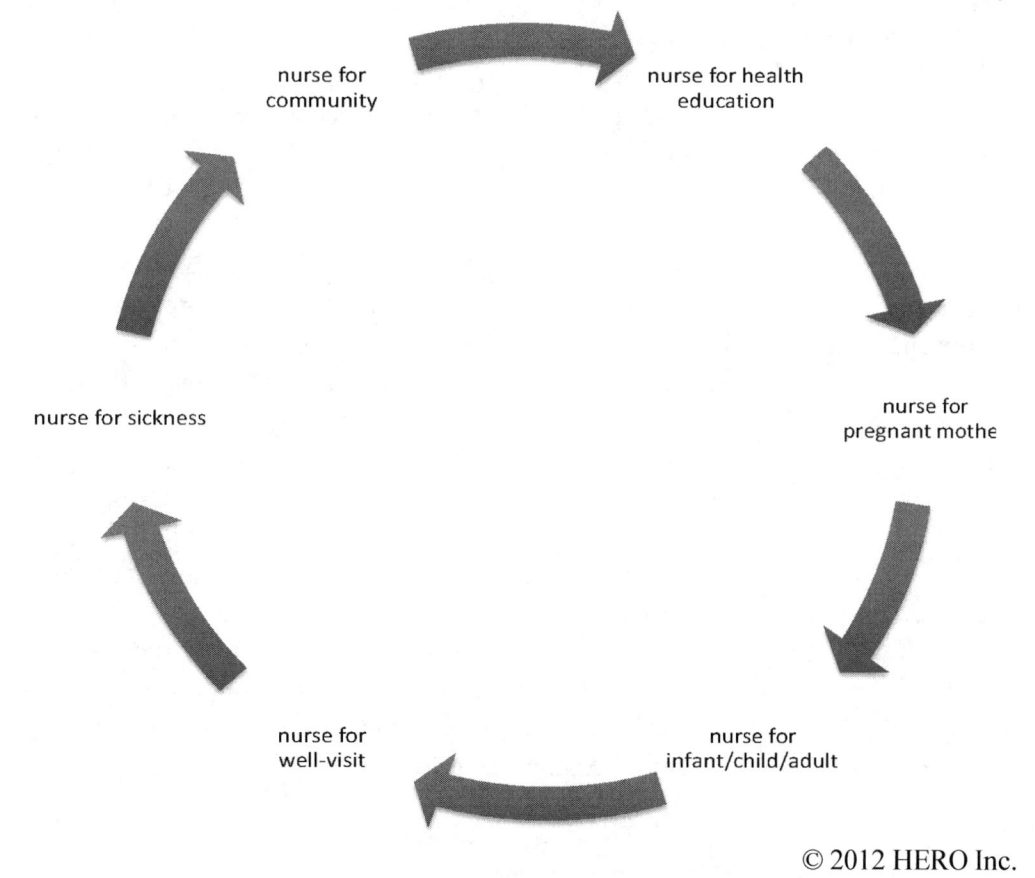

© 2012 HERO Inc.

Figure 1-2. Nurses Across all Sectors of Health

Since nurses are prominent across most healthcare settings, they are needed to make a successful impact on individuals and communities. Whether a nurse first addresses a community through a health promotion campaign, happens to be a mother who volunteers in the school setting, or casually provides health tips to her peers, nurses are well-educated, skilled providers, with the ability to lead to effective change.

As in any health setting, nurses play a crucial role. In clinical practice, nurses begin their training by learning to help patients ambulate and maneuver, and by assisting patients with range of motion, toileting, bathing, and more. Subjectively, nurses know that, at some point, they will need to call in another nurse to use the hydraulic lift to move a large patient, or at least receive some support with a large patient during a trip to the restroom. Whether nurses in clinical practice have viewed caring for an obese patient as a logistical challenge or not, nurses must be aware of how the increasing prevalence of obesity will challenge nursing care and the overall health of our patients.

The challenge for nurses is how to communicate this effectively to patients. We must be sensitive, yet we have to educate patients to understand the significant, yet highly preventable, effects of obesity.

Nurses must recognize that many people will:
1. Not recognize that they have a weight problem
2. May recognize a weight problem, but not recognize they have a risk of further health problems
3. Recognize these issues but not know how to make changes

By exploring the patient's knowledge and perception of his or her overall health, the nurse can better educate the patient on how to adopt small (but significant) measures to slowly improve health and reduce risk factors. Nurses can help dispel certain health myths, which will make patients more self-aware. This may lead to better understanding of the basic principles of nutrition and fitness, which will help the patient understand the need to prevent/reduce obesity or improve health, even if weight loss is not achievable in the short term.

Similarly, nurses must explore their own perception and judgments about obesity and health. Psychological research has demonstrated that even healthcare providers can react negatively to overweight and obese patients. Shorter appointment slots, little focus on obesity issues, and negative attitudes have been demonstrated by physicians caring for overweight and obese patients (Puhl et. al., 2005), which adds an additional burden. When patients perceive judgment by the provider, embarrassment and avoidance ensues.

With the significant increase in the number of patients who are overweight or obese, nurses must have a greater basic understanding of obesity in order to educate their patients without bias towards these patients. Further research by Puhl demonstrated that people have improved attitudes toward people who are obese when they perceive that others around them have more favorable attitudes toward obese people (Puhl, 2005). Thus, as a professional group, nurses should demonstrate positive attitudes, and understand the challenges that contribute to obesity. Then, as patient advocates, nurses can help their peers reduce surrounding bias and maintain a positive outlook, and reinforce to their patients that even subtle changes can have a dramatic effect. Helping others help themselves will promote an understanding that even minimal health changes are a progression to optimal health and wellbeing. In an effort to promote health, educate patients about obesity and health risks, always keep in mind what your role as a nurse should be. Create your own nursing acrostic or use ours, as a reminder of your role:

NURSE Acrostic

N: Nurture --- nurses show compassion and concern

U: Understand --- nurses listen and hear the patient's problem

R: Responsible --- nurses are licensed, ethical, and responsible for appropriate actions

S: Strategize --- nurses can develop a care plan to incorporate the many needs

E: Educate --- nurses guide and provide teaching tools to support the care plan

© 2012 HERO Inc.

Become a leader in the field, and discover that within your scope of nursing, your ability to encourage, teach and promote health can be endless.

> *"Nursing encompasses an art, a humanistic orientation, a feeling for the value of the individual, and an intuitive sense of ethics, and of the appropriateness of action taken."*
> — Myrtle Aydelotte

References

Active Living Research (2011). Research Brief: The Potential of Safe, Secure, Accessible Playgrounds to Increase Children's Physical Activity. Robert Wood Johnson Foundation. Retrieved on 05/24/12 at http://www.activelivingresearch.org/files/ALR_Brief_SafePlaygrounds.pdf

Garrett-Wright, D. (2011). Parental perception of preschool child body weight. Journal of Pediatric Nursing. Oct;26(5):435-45. Epub 2010 Sep 17. Retrieved on 06/06/12 at http://www.ncbi.nlm.nih.gov/pubmed/21930030

HHS announces revised Medicare obesity coverage policy. News releases of the Centers for Medicare and Medicaid Services, Washington, D.C., July 15, 2004. Accessed 05/25/06 at http://hhs.gov/news/press/2004pres/20040715.html

Institute of Medicine (2012). http://www.iom.edu/Reports/2012/Accelerating-Progress-in-Obesity-Prevention.aspxDec;58(6):1521-41, xii. Retrieved on 05/23/12

McPherson, M.E., Homer, C.J. (2011). Policies to support obesity prevention for children: a focus on early childhood policies. Pediatric Clinics of North America. Retrieved on 05/23/12 at http://www.ncbi.nlm.nih.gov/pubmed/22093867

Mello, M.M., Studdert, D. M., & Brennan, T.A. (2006). Obesity – The New Frontier of Public Health Law. New England Journal of Medicine; 354:2601-2610: June 15, 2006. Retrieved on 05/29/12 at http://www.nejm.org/doi/full/10.1056/NEJMhpr060227

Pelman ex rel. v. McDonald's Corp., 237 F. Supp. 2d 512 (S.D.N.Y. 2003), refiled as 2003 WL 22052778 (S.D.N.Y. Sept. 3, 2003), vacated in part, 396 F.3d 508 (2d Cir. 2005), remanded, 396 F. Supp. 2d 439 (S.D.N.Y. 2005).

Puhl, R.M., Schwartz, M.B., & Brownell, K.D. (2005) Impact of Perceived Consensus on Stereotypes About Obese People: A New Approach for Reducing Bias. Health Psychology, 517–525. Young-Hyman et al. (2000) entitled "Care Giver Perception of Children's Obesity-Related Health Risk: A Study of African American Families

World Health Organization (2011). SIXTY-FOURTH WORLD HEALTH ASSEMBLY, May 24, WHA64.7. Retrieved on 06/06/12 at http://apps.who.int/gb/ebwha/pdf_files/WHA64/A64_R7-en.pdf

World Health Organization. Definition: Nursing. Retrieved on 06/06/12 at http://www.who.int/topics/nursing/en/

Young-Hyman et al. (2000) entitled "Care Giver Perception of Children's Obesity-Related Health Risk: A Study of African American Families

Chapter 2
Obesity & Determinants of Health

Within the scope of any nursing care, nurses learn to assess how chronic illness, mental status, and body functions affect patients and their ability to ambulate, recover, eat and perform activities of daily living. To fully understand the implications of obesity and health, nurses must further explore topics of exercise, nutrition, illness, sleep, environment, family, smoking and alcohol use, in relationship to the patient's weight and size.

> Chapter 2 Objectives:
> 1. Illustrate why nutrition and weight are important
> 2. Summarize the relationship between health and physical fitness
> 3. Identify health conditions related to obesity: heart disease & diabetes
> 4. Explain how obesity relates to sleep and genetics

In Chapter 1, we discussed an individual's *perception* of health and how obesity affects public health. In this chapter, we use Healthy People 2020 as a basic guide to understand how leading health indicators are associated with health. So, what are the main determinants of health? The U.S. Department of Health and Human Services originally developed the Healthy People health promotion and disease prevention program in 1979 as a tool to set goals for the following decade. The program has been updated in 1990, 2000, 2010, and 2020 (for this decade). With over 42 target areas, and 600 objectives, this federal program provides important goals and target areas for health. We will use this tool to examine obesity in relationship to health status as a whole.

The complex issues of obesity and the consequences to the health of the individual if left untreated are staggering. Fighting obesity, losing weight, and improving health must be considered for overall health promotion. As a potentially long-term and life-threatening process, obesity must be *prevented* before it affects multiple body systems. Thus, understanding the determinants of health that relate to obesity is pertinent to obesity prevention and strategies.

Healthy People 2020 explains quite simply that nutrition and weight status are important to maintain health. Proper nutrition is essential for growth and development of children, as we will explore throughout the guide. And a healthful diet and proper weight are essential for all Americans to reduce conditions including, but not limited to:

- Overweight and obesity
- Heart disease
- High blood pressure
- Type 2 Diabetes
- Some cancers

Keeping in mind that there is a wide degree of variability among specific determinants of health for each *individual* and even each age group and race, Healthy People 2020 offers *guidelines* only, and not rules. It is the responsibility and within the scope of the nurse to use his or her own clinical acumen to successfully assess and synthesize how the individual patient can best meet health guidelines. To assist in this process of identifying health determinants, we explore the main categories including nutrition, physical activity, sleep, heart health, and diabetes.

Diet, Nutrition, and Obesity

Healthy People 2020 promotes a healthful diet and healthful weight by encouraging Americans to eat a variety of nutrient-dense foods, such as whole grains, fruits, vegetables, lean protein, and low-fat milk and dairy products. A healthy diet is also considered to be one with low intake of fats, trans fats, salt, sugar, and alcohol. A proper diet should also limit caloric intake to meet caloric demand (HHS & USDA, 2005). There is an assumption that an obese person cannot be malnourished, but nurses must consider *what* people eat, and not only *how much*. Many of us have cared for patients with a history of alcoholism who have been prescribed multivitamins to replace those vitamins and minerals depleted by alcoholism. Recognizing that size is not purely a symbol of health, the fact that a person of healthy size could eat less healthfully than their obese counterpart must also be considered.

Nurses must further appreciate that many determinants affect how and what our patients eat. Consider a few factors that influence nutrition and diet:

- Access to healthy foods
  - Availability of food pantries
  - Access to fresh fruits/vegetables
  - Mobility – ability of the patient to walk, drive, or use public transport to get to a store

- Cultural beliefs about foods (as we will explore in the next chapter)
    - Home environment, caretakers, support persons
    - Value placed on eating healthful foods
- Work or school schedule
    - Shift work (especially overnight) can hinder typical routines
    - School schedule and meals at school
- Food habits and social context
    - Purchase of fast-food versus home cooked meals
    - With whom does your patient typically share meals?

Taking into consideration the variability that may result from the above factors for each unique individual, we still need a basic guide to understand what a proper and healthful diet (regardless of overweight, underweight, or obese status) should consist of. We use the USDA Guidelines, founded on evidence-based research, to determine appropriate guidelines for all Americans.

The key components of the USDA's Choosemyplate.gov plan are:

Half the grains we eat should be whole grains

It would be unrealistic to tell people to eat *only* whole wheat breads or whole grain foods (brown rice instead of white rice), so an achievable goal is that half the starchy foods we consume should be whole grain. Read food labels and search for "100% Whole Grain" bread, which has more fiber.

Add More Vegetables

Make half your plate vegetables. Most vegetables are so low in calories that you can have a much greater *volume* of food for *more nutrients*, with less fat and fewer calories. Fresh or steamed vegetables are the best for you, though frozen or canned vegetables can be used as well. Washing canned vegetables can help reduce some of the sodium. Dark, leafy greens are very high in vitamins and are a better choice than lighter greens like iceberg lettuce.

Make Half Your Plate Fruits and Vegetables

A variety of colors and types of fruits and vegetables offer a variety of vitamins and minerals. Berries, such as strawberries and blueberries, are low in calories while high in antioxidants and vitamins.

Eat and Drink More Non-Fat and Low-Fat Dairy Products

"Skim the fat" to lower fat or non-fat dairy products. For instance, plain yogurt can be substituted for sour cream when cooking. Cream cheese and butter are not considered dairy products (as they are high in fats and oils).

Limit Salt and Sodium

Sodium increases high blood pressure. Eating more fresh foods, and foods prepared at home, can help reduce sodium and salt intake. Trying new condiments (vinegar, lemon juice, and spices) instead of salt can help lower sodium while adding flavor.

Limit Alcohol

Consuming more than one alcoholic beverage a day may increase the risk of various cancers. Please drink responsibly.

In reality, dietary recommendations are seldom followed consistently, even though many people may have a basic knowledge of food groups. Even the USDA struggles with how to balance food policy with the politics of the food industry and the needs of its citizens. Only recently have policies changed so that food policy is nutrient-based rather than "food based." Politics aside, people in America will eat what is readily available and cost-effective. With that in mind, we will examine a few striking differences between various world cultures in Chapter 3.

Obesity and Physical Activity

We know that nutrition and physical activity often go hand in hand, as they are clearly and inextricably linked. Remember that we must eat and consume nutrients for energy, and we expend energy through physical activity. Thus, the appropriate balance of energy intake and expenditure must always be considered. We must, therefore, fully explain the relationship between the two, and how an imbalance can contribute to obesity. Caloric intake is too high for most Americans, but over-exercising is also not an appropriate quick fix. Therefore, we explore guidelines to balance physical activity with caloric intake and promote overall health.

The Centers for Disease Control and Prevention (CDC) recommends that, for substantial health benefits, adults engage in 2 hours and 30 minutes of moderate to intense exercise a week; or 1 hour and 15 minutes of intense to vigorous exercise a week (PART IV will detail programs for your patients). Adding muscle strengthening exercises to your patient's regimen twice a week can result in additional health benefits (CDC, 2008).

Later in this book, we explore appropriate fitness activities for children, adults, individuals with disabilities and older adults. Just as we considered factors that affect nutrition and diet, we must know how multiple factors affect our patient's tendency or ability to engage in physical fitness.

- Environmental factors
  - Availability of sidewalks
  - Safety of neighborhoods
  - Climate and terrain
  - Availability of bicycles and sporting equipment
  - Public and private health facilities and their cost
- Social factors
  - Self-esteem and supportive environment (especially among females)
  - Cultural value of fitness and exercise (which we explore in the next chapter)
- Fear of Injury
  - The benefits of physical activities outweigh the risk, though safety must be considered (CDC, 2008)
  - Mobility and agility of the individual
  - Use of appropriate clothing and equipment
- Physical factors
  - Chronic illness
  - Respiratory function (in the case of patients who smoke or have asthma or pulmonary disease)
  - Prior experience and skill with fitness

The USDA, CDC, and Healthy People 2020 are all valuable and evidence-based tools you can print from or refer patients to, as a reminder of why physical activity is essential for better health. Using simple language, Healthy People 2020 explains how and why physical fitness can improve health for people of all ages, stages, and ability. Physical activity has demonstrated the ability to reduce the risk of following:

- Early death
- Heart disease
- Stroke
- High blood pressure
- Type 2 Diabetes
- Some cancers
- Falls
- Depression

The CDC successfully provides separate guidelines for different stages of life. For example, young adults, such as college students, have unique health determinants that can be easily and freely accessed. Referring young adults to informational sites like the CDC's site (cdc.gov/features/collegehealth) may encourage students to get regular checkups, get 2.5 hours of fitness a week, and follow a healthy diet. The CDC, like the American College Health Association, maintains healthy eating and activity as the top priorities:

- Improve eating habits and be active
- Avoid fatigue and sleep deprivation
- Maintain mental health
- Avoid substance use
- Have healthy relationships and prevent violence
- Prevent sexually transmitted diseases
- Quit smoking

*Notice also that the CDC lists *sleep* as the second priority. The sleep patterns of young adults are often inconsistent and fluctuate depending upon their course schedules, study habits, work schedules and social lives. This leads us to further explore how sleep and obesity are linked.

Sleep and Obesity

The CDC lists *sleep* as the second health priority for young adults, and the need for adequate sleep across all ages is well documented. One study on the sleep habits of incoming university students in Taiwan demonstrated that 54.7%

of students were classified among the "poor sleep quality" group, which was significantly associated with being an undergraduate, a female student, having less social support, higher neuroticism, more time on the Internet, and a tendency to skip breakfast (Cheng et. al., 2012).

Lack of sleep, in combination with poor eating (not to mention the prevalence of college alcohol consumption), can lead to poor school performance and less likelihood of remaining active. While there are plenty of active and healthy students who "pull all-nighters," inconsistent and sometimes extreme college behaviors certainly have a tendency towards decreased participation in health promoting activities. Thus, there is an obvious need to educate young adults in order to promote better health. Encouraging regular health screenings is *crucial*.

Nurses must consider the developmental age and stage when assessing sleep needs for a patient, as the required amount sleep will vary greatly. We know that babies sleep for the majority of the day, while older adults tend to require only a few hours a night, even without added mental health issues or dementia. Unfortunately, in a hospital setting, nurses and patients recognize that sleep may be temporarily impaired due to the nature of a hospital setting. But, especially when discussing health promotion in relation to obesity and general health, we must highlight the fact that sleep is a necessary component of overall wellbeing across a person's life span. From birth through childhood and adolescence, sleep is closely linked to growth and development and hormonal fluctuations within the body. According to healthypeople.gov, not only sleep duration but also the timing of sleep is crucial for metabolic, neurological and immunological function. Untreated sleep disorders and chronic short sleep (short sleep is defined as sleeping less than 6 hours a night) can increase the risk of the following:

- Heart disease
- High blood pressure
- Obesity
- Diabetes
- All-causes of mortality

In addition to these medical risks, lack of or poor sleep affects one's functionality at work and school, safety, and overall quality of life. Interpersonal relationships and family relationships can be greatly affected due to the depression, anxiety, and mood changes that may result from lack of sleep. Sleep disorders can affect people across all races, all socioeconomic states and all environments, and the effects of sleep disorders are widely overlooked. According to Healthy People 2020, 25% of adults in the U.S. report poor sleep health at least 15 out of

30 nights (Department of Health and Human Services 2012 and Van Cauter et al., 2008). Given the relationship between obesity, heart health, overall health at all ages, it would be wise to include sleep health among health promotion education. *Children and adults alike must not take for granted this basic necessity of life.* Treatment of sleep disorders, per se, is beyond the scope of this Guide, yet physical fitness and healthy eating have certainly influenced better sleep patterns. And the Appendix at the end of this book includes a Sleep Diary that can be a valuable tool for self-help sleep monitoring in an effort for the reader to better understand the issues at hand.

As with much of nursing care and implications of sleep on health, the difference between quality and quantity need be understood and differentiated. One study on obesity measured reported sleep quality and measured sleep time and eating habits among urban adults with a parental history of Type 2 Diabetes (Kilkus, 2012). While the timing of sleep did not demonstrate a significant change in eating (cognitive restraint, disinhibition, hunger, and uncontrolled and emotional eating), self-reported poorer quality of sleep did show a significant increase in hunger and uncontrolled eating. As we mentioned above, Healthy People 2020 stresses that poor health increases the risk of heart disease. And, as poor sleep and heart disease are associated with obesity, we must also explore heart disease as a significant health determinant.

Heart Disease

Heart disease remains the leading cause of death in adults and, in 2008, caused over 616,000 deaths in the United States (Centers for Disease Control, 2008). More than half of the deaths were among men, yet of the women who die each year, one in four women dies of heart disease (Centers for Disease Control, 2008). While there are many forms of heart disease, Coronary Artery Disease (CAD) is the leading type of heart disease, causing heart attacks in both men and women. Arteriosclerosis (also known as atherosclerosis), hypertension, and diabetes can all *contribute* to heart disease, though genetic predisposition clearly influences disease processes and susceptibility to risk factors.

According to the CDC, the best ways to *prevent* heart disease include:
1. Eating a healthy diet
2. Maintaining a healthy weight
3. Exercising regularly
4. Not smoking
5. Limiting alcohol consumption

Heart Disease and the Many Risk Factors

Heart disease is inextricably linked to obesity; we have discussed the best ways to *prevent* heart disease and now we will examine the risk factors. The following CDC chart shows the percentage of heart disease risk factors in U.S. adults from 2005 to 2008:

Risk Factor	%
Inactivity	53
Obesity	34
High Blood Pressure	32
Cigarette Smoking	21
High Cholesterol	15
Diabetes	11

Figure 3: Risk Factors for Heart Disease (2005-2008)
Centers for Disease Control and Prevention: Heart Disease Facts.
Reprinted with permission from the CDC.gov.

Note that the percentages in this table do not add up to 100% because, in 2003, approximately 37% of adults reported having two or more of the risk factors listed above.

A study by the American Heart Association (Hsia et. al., 2007) found that prehypertension was common across all races (around 40%), and was associated with an increased risk of heart attack, stroke, heart failure and cardiovascular-related death.

The CDC and National Health and Examination Nutrition Survey found that over the past decade, there has been an increase in adults ages 18-39 who take medication for hypertension (Gu et.al., 2006). Knowing that *obesity is a risk factor for hypertension, and hypertension is a risk factor for heart disease,* clinicians must focus on obesity prevention.

Diet and exercise are the standard first recommendations for how to "treat" cholesterol, hypertension, and even Type 2 Diabetes. Yet, in reality, there are no formal guidelines by which physicians decide at what point to give in to medication use when diet and exercise appear to fail. That is, it is widely up to the clinical judgment of the individual provider to determine whether or not diet and exercise will be successful, or if they should initiate medical treatment immediately. Patients become *more reliant and dependent* upon the individual physician and healthcare setting when they seek care only after illness or problems arise, rather than preventively. Oftentimes, patients do not realize *how and why* they should take the first and active approach to their own nutrition, activity, and wellness, to reduce the need for future health care. By advocating for oneself via improving health and nutrition, your patient can become his/her own health hero.

Knowing the guidelines of nutrition and fitness already covered in this Guide can help you arm your patients to choose foods that are lower in sodium, lower in cholesterol, higher in fiber, and higher in antioxidants, etc. Of course, we recognize that certain health determinants are not within our power (or our patients' power) to control or improve. But understanding even the minimal role our patient can take to reduce the likelihood of certain predispositions or health risks should be emphasized.

Genetics, Cancer, and Obesity

We have discussed environment, culture, and somewhat controllable and preventable influences on health. We must explore the genetics of health and determine if there is, in fact, a relationship between obesity and cancer. According to Healthy People 2020, cancer is one of the leading causes of death, second only to heart disease. Though it might not seem obvious, according to the National Cancer Institute, obesity is associated with an increased risk of many types of cancer, including the following:

- Esophagus
- Pancreas
- Colon and rectum
- Breast (after menopause)
- Endometrium (lining of the uterus)
- Kidney
- Thyroid
- Gallbladder

Just as the rate of diabetes is projected to soar by 2030, projections indicate that the current rising trends in obesity will lead to an additional 500,000 cases of cancer in the U.S. annually by 2030. Reducing every adult's BMI by even 1 kilogram (2.2 lbs) could significantly decrease that projected cancer rate by 100,000 cases per year. U.S. estimates from 2007 demonstrated that about 34,000 new cases of cancer in men (four percent) and 50,500 in women (seven percent) were due to obesity (National Cancer Institute 2012). This is significant and requires steady obesity prevention strategies.

There are various theories as to why obese people have an increased risk of cancer. It is possible that fat cells produce hormones, such as leptin, that affect cell growth. Fat cells may increase the amount of estrogen, which scientists have associated with an increased risk of breast and other cancers. Increased inflammatory responses and changes in tumor growth regulators in fat cells have also been associated with increased cancer risk. Given the significance of obesity and increased cancer risk, health education must include obesity *reduction and prevention* as an additional focus for cancer prevention.

There has been clear research to demonstrate a link between obesity and a variety of cancers and outcomes. A recent study of breast cancer survivors in rural Kansas demonstrated that obese breast cancer survivors had higher rates of recurrence and death compared to their normal weight counterparts. Given that rural women have higher rates of obesity, this study provided a weight loss program for cancer survivors. Results indicated significant weight loss, reduced blood sugars, and improved quality of life (Befort, 2011).

An article by Bracci (2012) explores the biochemical and genetic link of obesity to pancreatic cancer. Obesity is considered a "modifiable risk factor" for pancreatic cancer, one of the cancers with the poorest outcome. Similarly, diabetes is linked to higher risk of pancreatic cancer. Given that rates of obesity and diabetes are on the rise, in theory, reducing obesity and diabetes, could potentially reduce pancreatic cancer risk or improve outcomes.

In addition to understanding the associations between obesity and cancers, and increased risk factors for both, geneticists only now are learning the specific **genetic** expression of metabolic conditions. With the high incidence of obesity, diabetes and high cholesterol, understanding of the exact biochemical regulation of fat cells will become more and more important. At a molecular level, scientists have found a "master regulator," called leptin, which appears to regulate the fat cells and energy expenditure (Parachinni et al., 2005). As scientists learn more and more about the genetics of fat and obesity, healthcare providers can better understand the associations and risk factors for obesity and metabolic syndrome.

As nurses caring for patients who are overweight or obese, we clearly have little control over the genetics of their condition (as with any condition for which we care), and thus the modifiable environmental factors must be the focus of our efforts. How can we help our patients understand that, despite their higher risk factors (which they cannot control), there are still elements within their control to allow them to reduce their weight and eat well?

At a broader focus, how does race and ethnicity influence the epidemiology of obesity? No race or culture is immune to obesity, yet there are clear differential rates. We know that African-American and Hispanic groups have higher rates of childhood and adult obesity. And similarly, these groups demonstrate higher incidence and risk of hypertension, diabetes, and heart disease. As America becomes more diverse, with people of different nationalities and backgrounds, understanding the cultural perceptions of health will become more and more important to help educate Americans on lifestyle changes. If people do not believe they are overweight, obese, or at risk of the multiple complications associated with metabolic syndromes, will they be likely to take the necessary steps to improve their health?

Diabetes

There remains some confusion regarding the association between obesity and diabetes, since there are multiple forms or classifications of diabetes. Primarily, when discussing obesity and diabetes, this guide refers to Type 2 Diabetes, the most common form among adults (previously called Adult Onset Diabetes). In PART III, the specific classifications of diabetes will be discussed, but in this chapter, we explore the trends in the United States and how they relate to obesity. Statistics for people with diabetes between 1958 and 2009 show that the percent of the population with diagnosed diabetes has risen from under 1% to just under 7% in the United States. In 1958, there were approximately 1.5 million people with diabetes; today, that figure has risen to nearly 26 million people with diagnosed diabetes and another 79 million people in the U.S. with *prediabetes*. Unfortunately, many people with *prediabetes* are unaware of their increased risk of Type 2 Diabetes, heart attack, and stroke (CDC, 2012).

Diabetes has many severe complications, especially when left uncontrolled or untreated. Diabetes can lead to heart disease, heart attack, stroke, kidney disease and failure, blindness, diabetic neuropathy causing chronic pain, amputation, osteoarthritis, sleep apnea, gastroesophageal reflux disease (GERD), depression, and more. Nurses must understand, and help patients understand, that obesity increases the risk of having Type 2 Diabetes. While patients might not know the direct implications of becoming or being obese, a clinical condition, such as diabetes, might be of greater concern and be the needed impetus to encourage lifestyle changes for better health. Further still, nurses should recognize how, even aside from the added risks of chronic illnesses related to obesity, diabetes can be extremely debilitating, which makes certain lifestyle changes even more difficult to implement.

Projected future statistics for adults with diabetes are astounding, but are not completely surprising given the increase in the number of overweight and obese children and adults. An awareness of diabetes now must be one of our health education priorities. Just as we monitor blood pressure for heart disease, diabetics must have blood sugar monitoring (both fasting and hemoglobin A1C). Because the outcome and success of treatment for diabetes is largely related to the overall health of the person, nurses must be well versed in the general care of a diabetic patient.

According to Healthy People 2020, only 56.8 % of adults aged 18 years and older with *diagnosed* diabetes stated they received formal diabetes education at any time (age adjusted to the year 2000 standard population). Given the significant effect of diabetes on lifestyle and health status, along with the many complications and morbidities, diabetes education must be a priority.

All of these conditions, even in isolation, can be debilitating to an individual, but obesity further increases the risk of such conditions. While heart disease and cancer are the top two causes of mortality and morbidity during the adult years, so many conditions that ail the adult population are linked to obesity, which thus, directly or indirectly, causes morbidity and mortality in adulthood.

References

Befort, C.A., Klemp, J.R., Austin, H.L., Perri, M.G., Schmitz, K.H., Sullivan, D.K., & Fabian, C.J. (2011). Outcomes of a Weight Loss Intervention Among Rural Breast Cancer Survivors. Breast Cancer Res Treatment. Retrieved on 05/23/12 from http://www.ncbi.nlm.nih.gov/pubmed/22198470

Bracci, P.M. (2012). Obesity and Pancreatic Cancer: Overview of Epidemiologic Evidence and Biologic Mechanisms. Molecular Carcinogenics, 53-63.

Centers for Disease Control (CDC), (2008). National Physical Activity Plan, Physical Activity For Everyone. How Much Physical Activity Do Adults Need? Retrieved on 06/07/12 at http://www.cdc.gov/physicalactivity/everyone/guidelines/adults.html

Centers for Disease Control (CDC), (2008). CDC, Behavioral Risk Factor Surveillance System. Division For Heart Disease and Stroke Prevention, Heart Disease Death Rates 2000-2006. Retrieved on 06/10/12 at http://www.cdc.gov/dhdsp/data_statistics/fact_sheets/fs_women_heart.htm

Centers for Disease Control (CDC), (2012). Diabetes and Data Trends. Retrieved on 06/07/12 at http://www.cdc.gov/diabetes/statistics

Centers for Disease Control (CDC), (2012). National Diabetes Prevention Program. Retrieved on 06/10/12 at http://www.cdc.gov/diabetes/prevention/factsheet.htm

Cheng, S.H., Shih, C.C., Lee, I.H., Hou, Y.W., Chen, K.C., Chen, K.T., Yang, Y.K., Yang, Y.C. (2012). A study on the sleep quality of incoming university students. Psychiatry Research, Feb 17. [Epub ahead of print and retrieved on 02/27/12 at http://www.ncbi.nlm.nih.gov/pubmed/22342120

Department of Health and Human Services, Sleep Health. Retrieved on 06/08/12 at http://healthypeople.gov/2020/topicsobjectives2020/overview.aspx?topicid=38

Gebel, E. (2010). Diabetes Forecast Magazine. The Other Diabetes: LADA, or Type 1.5 Latent Autoimmune Diabetes in Adults is Gradually Being Understood. Retrieved on 03/03/12 at http://forecast.diabetes.org/magazine/features/other-diabetes-lada-or-type-

Gu, Q., Paulose-Ram, R., Dillon, C., and Burt, V. (2006). Antihypertensive Medication Use Among US Adults With Hypertension. Retrieved on 06/09/12 at http://www.cdc.gov/mmwr/preview/mmwrhtml/mm5520a14.htm

Hsia, J., Margolis, K., Eaton, C., Wenger, N., Allison, M., Wu, L., LaCroix, A., Black, H. (2007). Cardiovascular Disease in Women: Prehypertension and Cardiovascular Disease Risk in *Circulation*. 115: 855-860.

Johns Hopkins Medicine Health Alerts (2008). Johns Hopkins experts explain the difference between type 2 diabetes and Latent Autoimmune Diabetes of Adulthood (LADA).Retrieved on 02/29/12 at http://www.johnshopkinshealthalerts.com/reports/diabetes/1366-1.html

Kilkus, J.M., Booth, J.N., Bromley, L.E., Darukhanavala, A.P., Imperial, J.G., & Penev, P.D. (2011) Sleep and Eating Behavior in Adults at Risk for Type 2 Diabetes. *Nature Genetics*, 561-4. Retrieved 01/11/12 from http://www.ncbi.nlm.nih.gov/pubmed/21996663

National Cancer Institute at the National Institutes of Health (2012). Obesity and Cancer Risk. Retrieved on 04/19/12 at http://www.cancer.gov/cancertopics/factsheet/Risk/obesity

Paracchini, V., Pedotti, P., Taioli, E. (2005). Genetics of leptin and obesity: a HuGE review. *American Journal of Epidemiology*. Jul 15;162(2):101-14. Epub 2005 Jun 22.

Robbins, C.L., Dietz, P.M., Bombard, J., Tregear, M., Schmidt, S.M., Tregear, S.J. Lifestyle interventions for hypertension and dyslipidemia among women of reproductive age. Prev Chronic Dis 2011;8(6):A123. Accessed 12/11/11 at http://www.cdc.gov/pcd/issues/2011/nov/11_0029.htm

US Department of Health and Human Services (HHA) and US Department of Agriculture (USDA). Dietary guidelines for Americans, 2005. 6th ed. Washington: US Government Printing Office, 2005 January. Retrieved at http://www.healthypeople.gov/2020/topicsobjectives2020/default.aspx

Van Cauter, E., & Knutson, K.L., (2008). Sleep and the Epidemic of Obesity in Children and Adults. *European Journal of Endocrinology*, 159, Supplement 1, 59-66.

Chapter 3
Health & Food Culture Around the World

*"**Let your food be your medicine, and your** medicine **be your food."***
— Hippocrates

With the significant advancements in medicine and science since the time of Hippocrates, our civilization has changed greatly. Despite these great strides, modern society is plagued by a struggle between the scientific ability to live longer, and how to treat and live with the complications of environmental, social, and genetic factors influencing chronic illness and obesity. Though modern day life expectancies are higher that in ancient times, and fewer people die of simple infections; chronic illnesses affect people for *longer*. In light of the rising rate of obesity and how significantly this can compound chronic illness, there must now be a paradigm shift – a new focus on health education and how to best harness the resources of our modern day science and medical knowledge. In this chapter, we use anthropological evidence and cultural comparisons to examine the following:

Questions to consider:
1) How is health and food culture *today* different than in ancient times?
2) How is food culture in America different than across the globe?
3) How do different food and health cultures contribute to obesity?

Chapter 3 Objectives:
1. Explore the health and nutrition of ancient civilizations
2. Explain the evolving need for and use of federal food guidelines
3. Describe global trends in nutrition and health
4. Summarize the variety of food cultures existing within the United States

---

The Early Pyramids and Food

Looking back through time, we see that what is considered to be the epitome of health has changed drastically over the past number of centuries and decades, though some health issues remain unchanged. As this chapter explores changes in food habits, and changing in food pyramids, we look to the time of the Egyptian pyramids during that ancient civilization. Even 4,000 years ago, we see that certain knowledge of the body empowered people to follow a specific diet, use doctors of medicine, and gain support through religion or community. The ancient Egyptians were notorious for studying health and using some of the oldest techniques of surgery and medical science to help learn about the human body. Through the Egyptian mummies and embalming traditions, anthropologists and forensic scientists have learned much about the human body. Ancient Egyptians were known to have had a far more sophisticated knowledge of medicine than other cultures at that time.

To ready the body for mummification, Egyptians used tools and hooks to remove the brain through the nose. They removed internal organs as well, and thus had a well-versed knowledge of anatomy. Though Egyptians did not understand the exact physiology of the blood, they understood that blood and nerves were "channels" like the Nile River. They understood that, if the channels were not working correctly or were dry, they needed to be cleaned. There was even an awareness of infection and belief that the body was to be shaved and washed to keep a person healthy. Ancient medicine was also used in the form of animal and plant preparations for various treatments. Egyptians understood that some illnesses were treatable, while others were not.

Ancient Egyptians even understood the basics of nutrition and the need for moderation and balance far sooner than other more modern cultures thereafter (Dollinger, 2002). Based on archaeological findings, as well as human remains, we know that Egyptians and other civilizations as far back as 4,000 years ago ate diets rich in whole grains (mainly barley and wheat), meats, fish, fruits, vegetables, and oils (linseed and olive). Although severe drought leading to famine was not uncommon throughout history, during good times, the fertile soil of the Nile River banks offered nutrient rich farmland for growing grains and raising livestock. Archaeological finds reveal that goats, sheep and other livestock were eaten. However, certain animals were not part of the daily diet, as they were considered "unclean." This belief dates back to the Old Testament, and rooted itself in many of the laws of Kashrut (Kosher) and later Muslim cultures; in such cultures, meat from a pig is not considered fit for eating. (We will touch on this topic later).

Despite the availability of a variety of farmed and gathered foods, Egyptians did have a variety of nutritional deficiencies, including iron-deficiency anemia. This is evident by examining the bones of exhumed skulls and their eye orbits. It is possible that iron deficiency in this case was due to a diet high in grains and lower in protein than contemporary diets.

We know that ancient civilizations clearly had better diets (comprised of nuts, grains, meats, and vegetables) than many contemporary civilizations, but we also know that what we eat is not the only factor of health. Ancient cultures, by necessity, remained hard working manual laborers, with few exceptions.

The women were gatherers and tended to the children and the home, with no luxuries to minimize their work. The men were either hard laborers (building pyramids, tombs, and such) or rode horses, ran, hunted or walked incessantly.

Yet despite their better food and active lifestyle, we know that the Egyptians, as well as other ancient civilizations, had a significantly lower life expectancy than today. This is because contemporary Western medicine has extended life expectancy largely due to the use of antibiotics, decreases in traumatic injuries, and the use of heart medications.

In the U.S., it is safe to say that (despite a recession and current political debates regarding health policy) we have better health resources than ever before. Food, fitness, and health must be key components in showing the populace how health education can lead to *healthier* longer lives, free of illness and obesity. We point out here that, yes, modern medicine can treat infection, cure some conditions, mass produce foods and medicines, and use advanced technology, yet we have forgotten some basic elements of healthy living. Before we delve into food culture of other countries, let us look at the USDA recommendations to see how they have changed, yet how they maintain their basic foundation. It is this foundation of eating basic ingredients of grains, fruit, vegetables, and lean meats that really has not changed so much over time, even since ancient Egypt. But, while the recommendations have not changed so significantly, in practice and reality, it has become harder and harder to follow these guidelines.

Evolving "Food Pyramid" and Dietary Trends

Now skip forward two thousand years, and travel westward to the United States, where the need for food safety and health in the early 1900s helped structure the USDA as the federal program to maintain food safety and nutritional health. Over the past century, nutrition recommendations have changed somewhat (mostly in the graphical depiction) while still maintaining similar key components, which we should still follow today. The role of the US in providing those guidelines has shifted according to the times. In 1894, the USDA issued the first dietary recommendations for Americans, but it was not until 1916 that the first USDA book was published, *Food for Young Children* (Hunt, 1916). At that time, food categories were separated into 5 groups: milk and meat, cereals, vegetables and fruits, fats and fatty foods, and sugars and sugary foods. The author wrote that a child should receive at least one food from each group to receive sufficient nutrition, and the serving sizes depend on the age of the child. Photographs of plates of foods were included, with descriptions of their contents to help guide parents to understand the basic needs. Simplicity and variety of foods, ease of preparation, and good taste were all accounted for. The nominal use of sugars and fats were described too. Using some butter and oil was fine, though deep-frying or "scalloping" was not the preferred way. Even in 1916, before medical advances like the discovery of penicillin and infection control (in 1928), a fairly accurate foundation of nutrition was in development. Perhaps because the concepts of basic nutrition seem so simple, nutrition does not get the notoriety that other concepts in health do.

Yet the USDA continued to develop guidelines and roll with the times, even under duress during World War II, when the USDA presented guidelines according to cost, to enable people to eat according to budget. In 1943, the "Basic 7" food groups *(see Figure 3-2)* were introduced to highlight essential foods, and how to incorporate them into breakfast, lunch (or supper) and dinner (USDA National Agricultural Library, 2012). The USDA again revised guidelines, and used the "Basic 4" *(see Figure 3-3)* between 1956 and 1979. This included what we know as the common food groups: Dairy, Meat, Fruits and Vegetables, and Breads and Cereals (USDA National Agricultural Library, 2012).

Interestingly, the idea of a "food pyramid" (*matpyramid* in Swedish) was first published by the Swedish National Board of Health and Welfare in 1974, and included a base with grains, potatoes, margarine, and milk; fruits and vegetables above; fish, meat and eggs at the top (Coop, 1972). This pyramid, maintaining a close resemblance, was adapted by the USDA and later become the 1992 Food Guide Pyramid. To view images of the 1992 and 2005 USDA Food Guide Pyramids, visit CDC.gov.

While the USDA food charts have changed dramatically over the years, as food policies change, the illustrations still serve as reminders of an overarching guideline and message to send to our patients. While past charts may have been more intuitive (the illustration used today misses an opportunity to better teach children what food categories include), one can still use whatever is the easiest option for educational purposes.

NOTE: The HERO program taught kindergarten students using the Pyramid chart *(see Figure 3-1)*, but found that, with young children, the illustration was entirely unintuitive and did not help the children learn the categories of food.

Fortunately, when we realized this near the end of our pilot program, the guidelines had changed. In our experience, the USDA Plate depiction *(see Chapter 7, Figure 7-1)* is more understandable than the 2005 pyramid, though there still is a missed opportunity to provide photos of foods that could be more easily translated and comprehended by young children. Perhaps in another decade or so, the USDA guide will revert back to the food pyramid, which intuitively reminds us of Maslow's Hierarchy of Needs, with the greatest needs at the base.

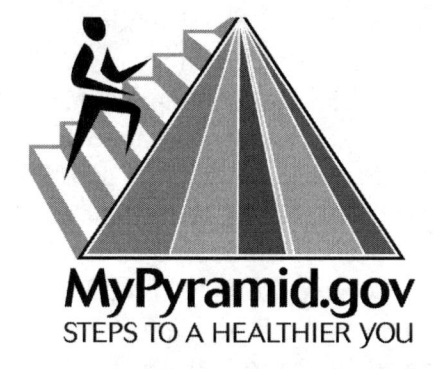

Figure 3-1. USDA "My Pyramid" (2005)
Reprinted with permission from the USDA.

Global Trends in Nutrition and Health

To examine basic trends in health around the world, we need to look at the statistics from the World Health Organization (WHO). The World Health Organization describes the growing global obesity epidemic as "globesity" (2102). As malnutrition has notoriously been the great public health concern across the globe and remains a leading cause of health loss (most for children under age five), obesity is paradoxically rising even among underdeveloped countries (World Health Organization, 2012).

WHO compares communicable illnesses, non-communicable illnesses, and injuries of various populations through various world regions to use statistics as a way of measuring and improving health trends. The burden of disease and statistics show that, while the mortality rates are clearly higher in undeveloped countries where poverty rates and hunger rates are higher along with lower access to care than in the Americas; some trends are beginning to shift (WHO,

2012). Overweight and obese people have become more pervasive, which is surprising among populations that typically were under-nourished. The burden of disease from obesity (and related mortality) is higher among high income countries, and is equally distributed among adults over age 60, and under age 60 (Lopez, et al., 2006). While mortality is greater from malnutrition in lower income countries, mortality from high blood pressure and obesity is higher in higher income countries (Lopez et al, 2006).

According to WHO, the preventable risk factors that influence morbidity and mortality throughout the world include "unsafe water and lack of sanitation; use of solid fuels in households; low birth weight; poor infant-feeding practices; childhood under-nutrition; being overweight or obese; harmful consumption of alcohol; use of tobacco; and unsafe sex."

Whereas obesity was rare among impoverished populations, westernization and changing eating trends are taking a toll on more and more subgroups across the world. Now, with the global obesity epidemic, we will see more countries modifying and adapting a national model of health, just as the U.S. borrowed from the Swedish. With so much World Wide Web information easily obtainable, those in search of health knowledge might find a clutter of computer-based information. Encouraging patients to use the federal guidelines can be a good starting point for health information. Though political to a point, the federal guidelines tend to have an evidence-based approach. Even looking to federal programs by other nations can provide added information. For an example, *(see Figure 3-4)* the healthy eating chart of the United Kingdom. We include this to show how the essential message is the same, as it offers similar services and education to their country. Thus, when starting an information and web-based search, even the national guidelines of other countries might offer more evidence-based support than computer health sites.

American Culture and Foods

We know America as the "melting pot" of many cultures, and thus America has a reputation for having many cultures melded together without a true defining culture of its own. America is famed for apple pie, hot dogs, hamburgers, pizza, and chicken nuggets.

Foods that originated elsewhere often take on a whole, new American way of preparation. A hot dog, which is not unlike German and Swiss frankfurters, has been dipped and batter-fried to become the American corndog. Still a carnival mainstay, corndogs are a common entrée in today's child meals at restaurants and public school cafeterias. This means that carnival food, which once was an annual treat, now has become daily food for some people.

One cannot discuss American food without mentioning McDonald's®, the single largest influence on American dietary habits. The quintessential chain, McDonald's® has such an influence on people throughout this country that the Ronald McDonald House Charities® provide care to patients, while McDonald's® restaurants feed the patients, families, and hospital staff across the way. It is a vicious cycle.

And yet, the fast food chain cannot be all to blame. Movies such as "Super-Size Me" have clearly blamed fast food for America's obesity epidemic, yet America's culture of food runs much deeper than just McDonald's®. Even cooking shows that could easily use the opportunity to educate people, instead sensationalize food by offering shows like "Man Versus Food," where the host travels to various restaurants to beat such eating challenges as eating a 140-pound burger or the biggest burrito ever seen.

The food industry and corporate America largely influence what is served, even in schools and hospitals, where we have known captive and impressionable audiences. But the American culture of freedom and independence enables us to make our own choices. A school board may allow the sale of soda or sugared beverages to children to supplement money for the school, but our children and our patients must be armed with the knowledge to know why we should balance what we eat and drink, and to make good choices.

Greek and Mediterranean Culture and Foods

Medical research has shown that the traditional Greek diet, largely comprised of seafood and vegetables, is often the healthiest diet available. This diet, often called the Mediterranean Diet (or MD for short), reduces the risk of heart disease. The word Mediterranean conjures up images of bright blue water and fields of olive trees, which are symbolic of the traditional primary foods consumed throughout the area. Fish is a staple food in a Greek diet, caught fresh from the ocean and grilled; not frozen or battered and then fried in oil. Seafood is incorporated almost daily with red meat eaten sparingly. Fresh fruits, nuts and vegetables are abundant. Vegetables are grilled and flavored with spices rather than salt, and salads are topped with a simple mixture of olive oil and vinegar, no ranch or bleu cheese dressing in sight, with bread dipped in oil, not spread thick with butter or margarine. Though olive oil, fish and nuts have a relatively high fat content, it is a combination of the healthy monounsaturated fat and Omega 3, which have proven health benefits (Mayo Clinic Staff, 2012). The simple, fresh approach to traditional Mediterranean eating makes it a healthy one.

Unfortunately, with the world striving to Westernize, there has been a shift in eating patterns worldwide. A recent Greek study showed that, of school children between the ages of 10 and 12, over 29% of them are overweight, while 10-12% are considered to be obese. These are the highest rates yet to be demonstrated among the Greek population. Of the children monitored in this study, it seems that urban children had the highest rates of being overweight or obese. As the Greek population strays from the traditional Mediterranean Diet (MD), its overall obesity rates rise (Farajian et al, 2011).

Japanese Culture and Foods

Next, let's take a look at the country that has the lowest overall rates of obesity in the world – Japan. (3.2% rate of obesity compared to the United States' 30.6% (the highest in the world), according to OECD's 2005 Health Data). What can Americans learn from the Japanese that might help us in our fight against obesity?

Japan's lower obesity rates have been attributed to its traditionally high intake of fish and vegetables. The Japanese eat in a starkly different manner then the rest of the world and, if you dissect the ever-popular sushi into its main components, you essentially have the crux of the Japanese diet. Japanese food is meant for presentation and appreciation, so a lot of time goes into making small portions look like works of art. The portion of a Japanese meal is much smaller then that of a traditional Western dish, which contributes to a lower intake of calories. Plain brown boiled rice is a foundation of every meal, with rice also served at breakfast time. The brown rice contributes to a filling low calorie dish and, along with fresh vegetables (either boiled into a broth, grilled or eaten raw), constitutes a very healthy way of eating. The Japanese account for the highest intake of fish per person in the world. They eat fresh fish, grilled or partly cooked, which is a great source of Omega 3 oil, combined with rice and vegetables in modest portions to make an incredibly healthy diet. (Moriyama, 2005).

In fact, the Japanese are actually more worried about underweight children than they are about overweight children, if you pay attention to data from the Organization for Economic Co-operation and Development Health. According to the 2005 OECD Health Data, one study of 617 urban students in Japan tracked BMI for students who were obese or underweight. Interestingly, there were fewer students determined to be *obese* than *underweight* (63 students, 10.2% of the study, were found to be *obese*, while 84 students, 13.6% of the study, were found to be *underweight*, respectively) (Ge, 2011).

Obesity was detected earlier among boys (between the ages of 6-8) than among girls (where it tends to show up between the ages of 12-14). Underweight was detected at later ages, at 12-14 for boys, and 15-17 for girls. But, as Japan adopts more Westernized culture, the food trends may change, and then they may see increased rates of obesity.

> **NOTE:** In America, the incidence of obesity has been so high that BMI studies focus mostly on obesity and not on being underweight. Certainly, the rates are higher for obesity in the US than they are for being underweight.

Chinese Culture and Foods

China, throughout history, has been known for its rice, soybeans, and wide variety of cuisine. Despite the differences from region to region (as China is a huge country both in area and population), some things remain constant: meals rely on rice, vegetables, and a small amount of meat, unless the person in question is quite wealthy – in which case, there are a wider variety of foods available (Tannahill, 1988). In the first instance, the Chinese don't view food as calories in, or calories out, they think of food as simply nourishment to care for the body, eating just until their hunger is satisfied. The Chinese also view vegetables as a meal, not a side dish, like many Western countries do. A meal can simply be a plate of vegetables accompanied by a broth-like soup: low in calories, high in nutrients.

In current times, the diet has changed only in larger cities, where American fast foods have come into play. Perhaps this is why obesity rates, which remain low throughout rural China, have risen dramatically in the cities. And, although the obesity rates are relatively low in China, given the high population, about one fifth of the one billion obese people in the world are Chinese (Wu, 2006).

Due to the enormous population, health disparities are great. Malnutrition and poverty remain a public health problem, with high rates of anemia, iodine deficiency, and low food intake. The Chinese government recognizes that public health, food safety, and nutrition are closely linked to the socioeconomic development of the China.

Notoriously, food safety in China has been an issue. After the contamination of baby milk in 2005, the Chinese government developed a Joint Program, recognizing that a multidisciplinary approach is crucial for successful policy and intervention to improve nutrition and food safety. China also recognizes that intervention in schools can be an effective way to promote health education, and that food safety and adequate nutrition in schools are critical first steps (Luo et al, 2002).

In 1995, the Physical Health Law of the People's Republic of China was adopted to help set a national standard for improving the fitness and physical conditioning of the Chinese people (China Internet Information Center 1995). A 2001 national survey by China's State Physical Culture Administration, spanned 3 years and had a goal of determining the exercise habits across 31 provinces in China. The study indicated that nearly 40 % of the total population, aged between 7 and 70, exercise and more than 60 % of urban residents go to sports clubs for physical fitness activities. By the end of 2005, over 95 percent of students reached the National Physical Exercise Standard, and the goal for 2010 was to have 40% of people across the country exercising regularly.

Unlike in the United States, in China it is commonplace to see a park with older adults exercising on fitness equipment. Chinese society prioritizes health and fitness even well into old age, and government programs support an active lifestyle. In this way, China demonstrates how social focus on public health and fitness can help thwart the rise of obesity. Yet it is unlikely that the U.S. will adopt compulsory fitness policies in that same way.

While there are sometimes mandates for compulsory fitness at school, such as in Florida (150 minutes a week), American society as a whole does not have compulsory health and fitness programs. And even a mandated program may not be heavily enforced. Looking at various cultures, though, can be a guiding force to brainstorm and understand the successes and strategies used by other societies across the globe, and help translate those programs to American society.

French Food and the Epitome of European Cuisine

Many of the European regions ate a similar diet until they differentiated into nation-states in the early centuries A.D. Grains were a main staple and crop, and corn and potatoes were only used after their importation from the New World. French cuisine, some of the world's most elegant and rich food, took shape during the Middle Ages, when Paris was the hub of royalty and social distinction. Guilds (or associations) were formed that separated the hunters/farmers from the pastry chefs and prepared food providers. Skilled culinary chefs provided colorful presentations of food, and seasonal ingredients embodied the cuisine.

Today, French food remains flavorful, rich, and elegant. The French, well known for smoking cigarettes and drinking loads of wine and coffee, also have a reputation for eating small quantities of food, despite the decadence of cheese and wine. High-end French restaurants, to an American, have miniscule portions, compensated for by having such flavorful and elegant ingredients.

Despite this, the French are not immune to the dietary trends of the Western world. A study of over 1,000 French youth in 100 elementary schools found that **17.3% were overweight** (*Obesity*, 2010). And, interestingly, the consumption of wine by young adults has declined, while the consumption of fruit juices has increased. The result of this change is inconclusive as to its effects on obesity rates, though slow changes in eating habits may be noted.

Still, we see significant differences in eating habits. Meat is seldom part of a breakfast, unlike an American breakfast of bacon and eggs or sausage and biscuits. A typical French breakfast includes bread with jam or a croissant sometimes with chocolate, tea, or coffee. (Children drink hot chocolate.) The largest meal of the day is the midday lunch, often taking an hour or two of the day. Children rarely buy food in a cafeteria, and more likely bring a packed lunch. Dinners are often three-course meals that include wine and bread.

France has taken such a stance against foreign culture's infiltration into French cuisine that Burger King® has not been able to remain established in France (though McDonald's® still expands its offerings there). And, to demonstrate the policies that France uses to keep their culture's cuisine inviolate, *ketchup was banned in school cafeterias* (unless it is used on French fries, though fries are limited and provided only on a weekly basis). As quoted in the *Los Angeles Times* (Oct. 6, 2011): "France must be an example to the world in the quality of its food, starting with its children," said Bruno Le Maire, the agriculture and food minister. While a policy to ban a condiment seems extreme and likely would not occur in the US, the awareness of the causes of poor eating (such as high sugar, high sodium condiments) should be appreciated across all cultures.

African Culture and Foods

As Africa is the second-largest landmass on earth, it is not surprising that African foods vary significantly across all regions. With hundreds of different cultures and subcultures, the typical "diet" varies, though it has certain commonalities. Many African meals include a starchy food (cassava, yam, rice, plantains) with a stew (with or without meat) served atop them. Barley, corn, millet, rice and couscous are used in meals – whatever grain or base food is least expensive and can fill the most people. Northern Africa, influenced by Turks and Arabs, has adopted many spices, such as cardamom, mint, cinnamon, and cloves.

It is believed that West Africans received certain influences from the Americas, from Christopher Columbus, soon after he sailed to America. Chili and tomatoes were introduced to West Africa, and are still widely used today. West Africans clearly are now more influenced by American food, as they now eat more meat, along with higher fat and higher sodium foods than before.

South American Culture and Foods

To Americans, Mexico often predominates as the commonly thought-of South American country, perhaps due to its proximity and cultural influences of food across its border with the United States. Interestingly, Mexico is ranked as having the second highest rates of obesity, second only to the United States, with obesity of 26.2% of the population according to the OECD Health Data (2005). Because of this, too, perhaps many people tend to conflate the many cultures across South America, when really Mexico does not share the predominant diet of other South American countries. A Mexican culture of pork, fried foods, refried beans, and an abundance of starch (corn, wheat, rice products) contributes to Mexico's excess of calories, fat, and sodium, and high rates of diabetes, heart disease, and obesity. Other South American countries, like Chile, Honduras, and Brazil, have quite varied diets and their obesity rates are not as high. Yet, a journal article in 2001 (Uauy et. al) described how the industrialization of South American countries, and change from poverty to more wealth, have taken a toll of mortality from chronic illnesses. While infection rates have declined with industrialization, obesity rates and death from chronic illnesses like heart disease and diabetes have increased. In general, throughout Latin America, as income increases across a county, so does the obesity rate, especially among urban women (Uauy et. al, 2001).

In Brazil, a study of 5,100 school children found that rates of overweight and obese children were higher among children of higher socioeconomic status compared to poorer rural children; this was attributed to those children riding in a car to school instead of walking, and doing less manual labor. Overall, though, Brazilian rates of obesity for children were far lower than in the U.S., with obesity rates of 2.7% and 1.5% for girls and boys ages 6-18 respectively. In contrast to these relatively low rates of obesity for Brazilian children, the prevalence of obesity among men and women across the Caribbean were as high as 20% and 48%, respectively, even in 1995 (Guedes et. al, 2011). Since we cannot compare apples to oranges, we must recognize how different cultures, levels of poverty and education, and access to foods and healthcare all contribute to the rising trends of obesity throughout South America.

Jewish Culture and Kosher Foods

Even within the United States, different cultures, ethnicities, and food habits can affect food choices and health patterns. There are roughly 6 million Jewish people throughout the United States, around 6 million Jews living in Israel, and smaller populations throughout the rest of the world. Yet only 15% of the Jewish population eats Kosher, according to strict dietary law called *Kashrut*.

It is typically the Orthodox Jews (sometimes the Conservative and Reform Jews, as well) who follow the most stringent dietary rules. As with Muslims and Halal foods, Jews who eat kosher may not eat pig or pork products, nor may they eat shellfish or certain seafood. Animals that have the potential to be kosher (cows, lamb, chickens, ducks, goats) must still be slaughtered according to strict Orthodox Jewish law. Traditions and rules dating back thousands of years are still followed today. Milk or dairy foods may not be consumed together with meat foods, and there is a waiting period of usually 3 or 6 hours between eating meat before dairy can be consumed (this depends on ancestral tradition). The cattle and other mammals' meat must be soaked and salted to remove all the blood. The Pentateuch, or Five Books of Moses (included in the Torah), dictate the dietary rules governing kosher eating.

Many of the kosher rules originated to prevent animal cruelty and to insure cleanliness of food (including specific ways of slaughter to minimize pain to the animal and not eating birds of prey or bottom-feeding sea animals). Because of this, it is not surprising that 85% of people buying kosher foods are not even Jewish.

But it is important to understand that this code of religious dietary law *does not* preclude a person from eating poorly, eating unhealthful foods, or not being physically active. Jewish heritage has a long history of food strongly linked to culture and, as with many cultures, holidays revolve around the dining room table. With the Sabbath occurring on a weekly basis, there is a culture of rest and eating on the weekends. And many of the foods consumed at this time are high in salt (meat is saltier by virtue of the method of slaughter) and high in fat. While access to restaurant foods might be limited in a region without a preponderance of Jews and kosher restaurants, many foods brought into the home are processed in a way similar to that of other Americans. Even without McDonald's® and other fast food, obesity can ensue and increase the risk of diabetes, heart disease and cancers. In fact, as compared to any other ethnicity worldwide, Ashkenazi (those of Eastern European descent) Jews have the highest lifetime cancer risk. Note than not all Jews are restricted to Kosher diets, yet still they have a predisposition towards certain cancers. So, the implications of obesity on health and cancer, would also support the need for health promotion among this group of people (Lynch et. al, 2004).

Muslim Culture and Halal Foods

As with kosher foods, Halal foods also must not contain any pig or pork ingredients. The varieties of meat that are acceptable must be slaughtered according to Shari'ah (Islamic Law) and handled in a specific way, overseen by a Halal Muslim authority who monitors the process to ensure that Halal foods are not cross-contaminated with non-Halal meats and food products. Sometimes, vegetarian meals are selected in the absence of Halal certified meals, due to the absence of any meat products appropriate for consumption. Understanding the strict belief system of the Muslims, and helping to procure adequate meals, especially when caring for an in-hospital patient, is critical.

Summary

Over time, people living in various cultures have adapted to the food sources available to them. This is why the Chinese and Japanese (among others) learned to cook with little meat or dairy products; and why the Greeks eat fish and olive oil (they had many olive trees). Despite a cultural love of wine and cheese, even the French may have decided to use smaller portions of the rich foods – original – due to economic necessity (Tannahill, 1988). And other cultures continue to change eating patterns as they rise from poverty. Unfortunately, obesity continues to be a pandemic, with no cultural or economic boundaries.

One thing is certain: no matter what your culture, no matter what type of foods you eat, there remains a need to *balance* intake of food and calories with output by exercise and activity. Across many cultures and countries, we see how poverty levels, influences of westernized eating habits, and limited use of manual labor have all affected obesity rates in a complex way. The rising trend of obesity is consistently seen throughout the world, despite improved infection control, and deep-rooted food cultures that are not American in nature.

Despite many cultural and ethnic differences around the world, there remain some common factors. Preparing meals using whole foods, lean fish and meats (as do the Greeks, Japanese, and Chinese) can increase nutritional value and decrease fat. Eating a wide variety of foods including fruits, vegetables, spices, whole grains, and olive oils, as seen across many cultures, also seems to help. **Moderation** of intake of calories, fat, and salt, and **increase** in activity levels (regardless of *what* you eat or *how* you are active), remain key components in improving your overall nutritional health, regardless of your culture.

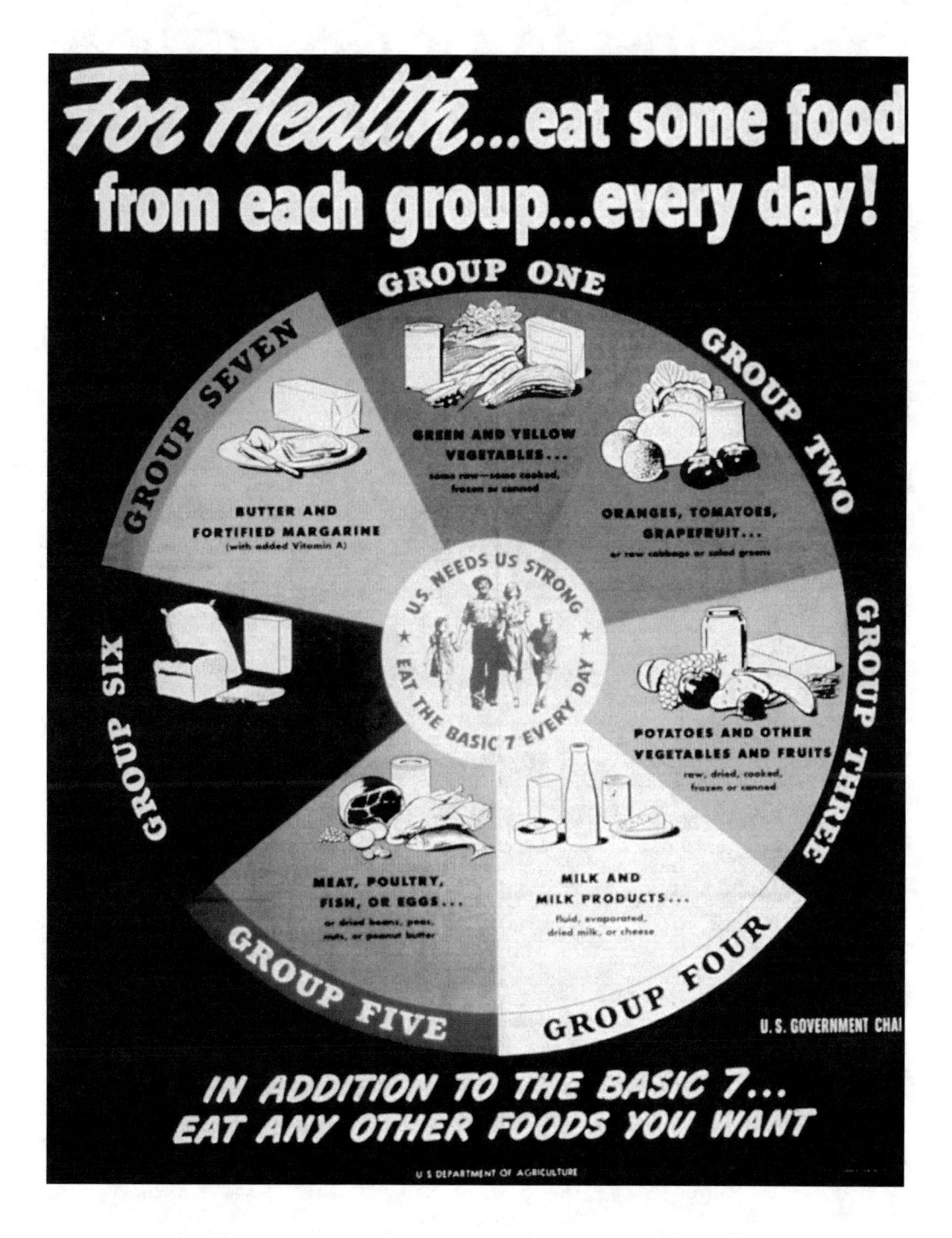

Figure 3-2. USDA "Basic 7" Food Guide Poster (1943)
Reprinted with permission from the USDA.

3: Health & Food Culture Around the World

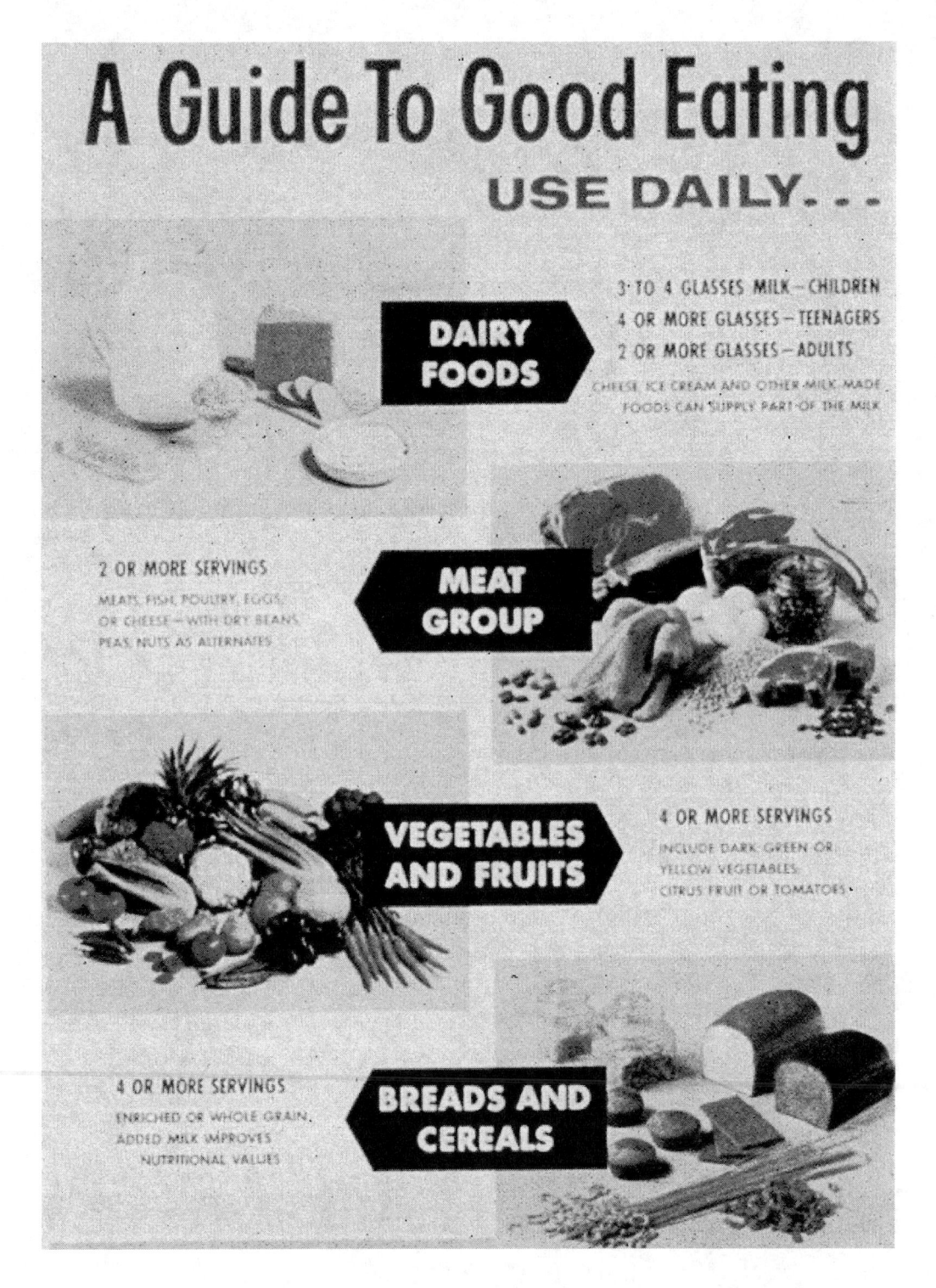

Figure 3-3. USDA "Basic 4" Food Guide Poster (1956-1979)
Reprinted with permission from the USDA.

48

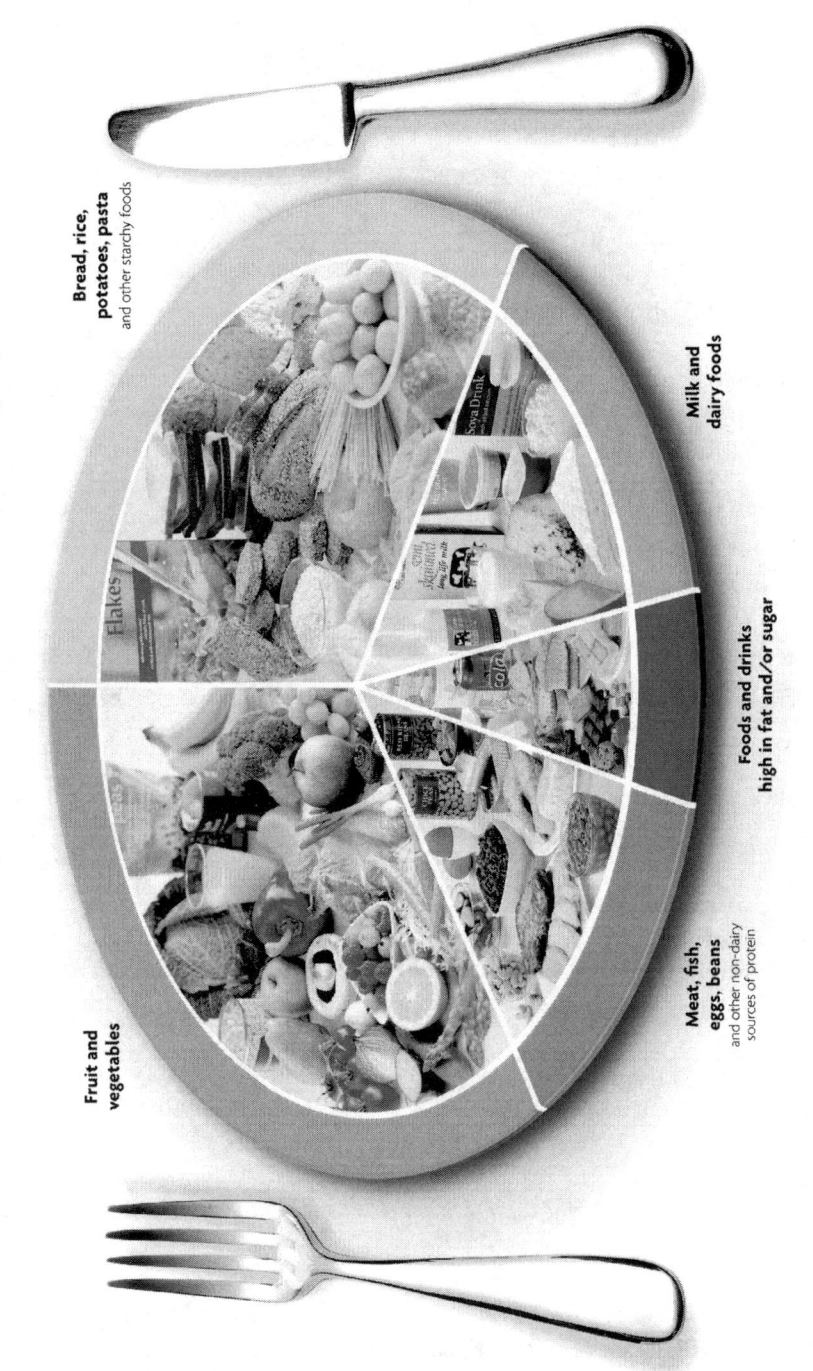

Figure 3-4. NHS Food Guide Plate
Department of Health in association with the Welsh Government, the Scottish Government and Food Standards Agency in Northern Ireland
Reprinted with permission from the National Health Service (NHS).

References

China Internet Information Center (2012) China Through A Lens. Retrieved 02/24/12 from http://www.china.org.cn/english/features/China2004/107193.htm

Coop (1972) Swedish Article Retrieved 05/10/12 from http://www.coop.se/Globalasidor/OmKF/Kooperativ-samverkan/Var-historia1/Tidslinjen/1960-19901/1973/KF-Provkok-lanserar-iden-om-basmat/

Farajian, P., Risvas, G., Karasouli, K., Pounis, G.D., Kastorini, C.M., Panagiotakos, D.B., and Zampelas, A. (2011). Very High Childhood Obesity Prevalence and Low Adherence Rates to the Mediterranean diet in Greek children: the GRECO study Aug;217(2):525-30. Epub 2011 Apr 13. Sourced from the Unit of Human Nutrition, Department of Food Science and Technology, Agricultural University of Athens, Iera Odos 75, 11855 Athens, Greece. Retrieved 05/08/12 from http://www.ncbi.nlm.nih.gov/pubmed/21561621

Ge, S., Kubota, M., Nagai, A., Mamemoto, K., & Kojima, C. (2011). Retrospective Individual Tracking of Body Mass index in Obese and Thin Adolescents Back to Childhood, *Asia Pacific Journal of Clinical Nutrition*, 432-7.

Guedes, D.P., Rocha, G.D., Silva, A.J., Carvalhal, I.M., Coelho, E.M. (2011). Effects of Social and Environmental Determinants on Overweight and Obesity among Brazilian Schoolchildren from a Developing region, *Rev Panam Salud Publica*. 2011 Oct;30(4):295-302.

Hippocrates Quote, retrieved on 05/5/12 at http://www.foodreference.com/html/qfood.html

Hunt, C. (1916). Food for young children, Published by U.S. Dept. of Agriculture in Washington, D.C., Retrieved 04/24/12 from http://archive.org/stream/foodforyoungchil00hunt#page/2/mode/2up

Instituto de Nutricion y Tecnologia de los Alimentos (INTA), Universidad de Chile, Santiago, Chile

Lopez, A., Mathers, C., Ezzati, M., Jamison, D.T., and Murray, C. (2006). Global Burden of Disease and Risk Factors: Disease Control Priorities Project, Washington (DC): World Bank; Retrieved on 07/17/12 at http://files.dcp2.org/pdf/GBD/GBD04.pd

Luo, J. and Hu, F.B., (2002): Time Trends of Obesity in Pre-School Children in China from 1989 to 1997, *International Journal of Obesity*, 26 553–58.

Lynch, H.T., Rubinstein, W.S., Locker, G.Y. (2004). Cancer in Jews: Introduction and overview. *Family Cancer*. 2004;3(3-4):177-92.

Mayo Clinic Staff (2012), Mediterranean Diet: Choose This Heart-Healthy Diet Option. Retrieved at Mayo Clinic Website 05/30/12 from http://www.mayoclinic.com/health/mediterranean-diet/CL00011/NSECTIONGROUP=2

Moriyama, N. & Doyle, W. (2005). *Japanese Women Don't Get Old or Fat*. New York: Delacorte Press, Random House.

Tannahill, R., (1988). *Food in History*. Penguin, London, England.

Uauy, R., Albala, C., and Kain, J. (2001) Obesity Trends in Latin America: Transiting from Under- to Overweight Retrieved 03/24/12 from http://wiki.dianebarrett.com/images/5/56/Obesity_Trends.pdf

United States Department of Agriculture (USDA), National Agriculture Library (2012). Retrieved 05/10/12 from http://www.nal.usda.gov/fnic/history/basic7.htm

Wang, Y., Mi, J., Shan, X.Y., Wang, Q.J., and Ge, K.Y., (2007). Is China Facing an Obesity Epidemic and the Consequences? The Trends in Obesity and Chronic Disease in China. *International Journal of Obesity* (London), 2007 Jan;31(1):177-88. Retrieved 06/09/12 from http://www.ncbi.nlm.nih.gov/pubmed/16652128

World Health Organization (2012). Controlling the Global Obesity Epidemic. Retrieved on 07/17/12 at http://www.who.int/nutrition/topics/obesity/en/

PART II: OBJECTIVE

In Part I, we learned about social health determinants of individuals and cultures in America and abroad. This first step was significant since a thorough patient assessment includes these background influences. Nurses must individualize their care by learning the context of that patient, and their specific needs, concerns, and problems. Now, as their next step (objective), nurses must identify specific objective data for that individual patient. Consideration of context (subjective) and the patient's baseline (history of objective data) of a patient is essential for successful clinical examination and judgment. Throughout all these steps, nurses must use keen communication and assessment to gather information pertinent to the patient "problem," namely obesity and/or the need for health maintenance. Nurses must keep an open mind, and understand the role of the nurse throughout all steps in the care process.

Part II examines actual identifiable and objective data, and obesity-related health conditions including diabetes and heart disease. Learning key factors related to a patient health assessment and review of systems is essential before understanding how to thoroughly conduct a physical exam. Astute clinical skills must be used, as obesity does not affect all people in the same way. The differences between adult and child health histories, and how to understand the added concerns for people with disabilities, will be discussed.

PART II Objectives:
1. Explain the importance of a patient health history and review of systems
2. Recognize clinical obesity and how to measure and monitor growth
3. Assess physical exam findings in obese and overweight patients
4. Support how underlying disability influences obesity
5. Illustrate the impact of obesity on diabetes and hypertension

Chapter 4
Health History, Review of Systems & Obesity

Although the health history, per se, would typically be classified within a subjective portion, we group this portion with physical examination and other objective data so that nurses can better understand the clinical and assessment process as a whole.

> Chapter 4 Objectives:
> 1. Explain how to conduct a health history and build patient rapport
> 2. Identify what characteristics to look for among adults and children
> 3. Determine what questions to ask during a Review of Systems

In lay terms, when we wish to gather information to address a specific issue, we must ask a few questions to put together a puzzle. Who? What? When? Where? Why? And How? Answers to these simple questions help establish a history and a context, and provide needed information to process the problem and enable a solution or resolution. In a similar way, nurses gather data (some subjective, some objective) via taking a health history and review of systems, then conducting a physical exam. While nurses may not have the time, authority, or position to conduct the full assessment, we must all be well versed in the total process. Translating the problem of "weight gain" into the questions a lay person might ask, we explore how easily we can obtain the data nurses need.

For instance, we see a child with a history of recent weight gain, and we ask:
- Who: the patient – age, gender, developmental stage, other illnesses
- What: the problem – complains of weight gain, chest pain, back ache, etc.
- When: onset of the problem – was the patient heavy as a child, young adult, etc.
- Where: more context – where is the weight gain
- Why: more context – has this happened before? Why does the patient think he has gained weight?

Remember that taking a **health history** is an important opportunity to ***build rapport with the patient*** before you examine him, but it also provides needed concrete information. It is the nurse's chance to assess the patient subjectively while the patient has the opportunity to do the talking. It is crucial at this point to be cautious and not put a patient on the defensive. Sensitivity, patience, and professionalism must be practiced for best history-taking. Learning about the patient, and taking the time to read body language, and understand cultural perspectives and health perceptions can help the nurse spare the patient intimidation and embarrassment during a vulnerable time. In a health history, we need to ask people questions about their body systems and any family history of illness, both physical and mental.

The exact manner in which the nurse conducts the Health History is at his or her own discretion, though practice makes this process easier. Remembering that eye contact, patience in awaiting responses, and sitting down with the individual (rather than standing) results in a warmer reception and will more likely elicit full responses. Below are the essential elements of the Adult Health History. Pay close attention to each NOTE that highlights issues specifically relevant to obesity and related issues.

Adult Health History:

Date of History: the Date is always essential for context and comparison

Identifying Data: Age, date of birth, occupation, religion

Source of History: Is the patient accompanied by family, friend, or interpreter? *If the patient is a child (over 5) or teen, they can still give a very good history.*

History of Prior Illness: Onset (when?), for how long? Any treatment already given?

Family History: Diabetes, hypertension, cancers, blood or bone disease, etc.

Allergies: Medication and/or food allergies. *What are the allergic effects? Itchiness versus anaphylaxis?*

Medications: Include over-the-counter (OTC) and herbal preparations

Alcohol/Tobacco/Drug Use: How often? Number of packs per day (ppd). Chewing tobacco (oral exam will be significant) or smokeless tobacco?

Remember that patients will often minimize their use of these. During the exam, the nurse should make a subjective note if a patient smells of alcohol or tobacco.

Diet: Include food restrictions, allergies, favorite foods and drinks and consumption of caffeinated beverages.

> **NOTE:** Notoriously, nutrition has been a subject often skimmed over by nurses and medical professionals, as the issue has been a concern of nutritionists in the medical setting (Müller, et, al, 2001). HERO zeroes in on nutrition as a highly necessary focus of a well-trained nurse, as **diet** so greatly influences the human body. The foods our patient typically eats can convey a wealth of knowledge about their overall health and risk of obesity and conditions including heart disease, diabetes, hypertension and more.

Exercise: Frequency and type of exercise. Typical mode of transportation. Limitations of exercise. Interest in exercise.

> **NOTE:** Similarly, exercise has not been a nursing concern other than mobility-related issues after surgery or due to illness or surgery. For instance, nurses learn about range of motion (ROM), the need to ambulate soon after surgery to reduce risk of blood clots and to avoid muscle atrophy. Exercise for prevention has not been a focus until now – due to the overwhelming prevalence of obesity across all ages.

Sleep Patterns: How many hours of sleep a night? Are naps taken? Medication for sleep?

> **NOTE:** Excessive number of hours slept can be an indication of depressive symptoms, or medication side effects. Few hours slept can be an indication of anxiety or stress, though often more typical with an older adult (Van Cauter, et al 2008).

Immunizations: Annual Flu vaccine? For women – vaccines for birth control or HPV?

> **NOTE:** For children, this is especially important, as immunizations are required to enter public school. There are parents who do not vaccinate their children due to fear of side effects and even development of autism (evidence for these concerns has not been medically proven, but this is beyond the scope of this Guide).

Psychosocial History: Includes elements that capture the overall wellbeing of the person. Daily Life, Significant Others, Religion, Occupation, etc.

All these elements greatly affect the person across all situations of health and illness. Who is their support person? Do they have one? Are they a caretaker of others?

Children's Health

First of all, we already may have some context for the child. Children are likely to be accompanied by an adult, and most likely are accompanied by their mothers. But you must not assume any relationships. Sometimes, an older adult with a child could be a parent, grandparent, step-parent, or foster parent ... the best approach is to ask, "How are you two related?" Remember that, as familial relationships are evolving with fewer nuclear families and more extended families, it is important to understand family dynamics to help understand the individual child and his or her family setting.

What are the major differences in taking a health history of a child? You need to know how to balance obtaining information from both the young patient and the caregiver. By age five, most children are fairly consistent in sharing how they feel. Though the nurse may well have two historians who may share details, your assessment of both the child and caregiver's body language is essential.

Child Health History:

Name and Nickname: Asking about a nickname is a good "icebreaker" for kids

Date of Exam: Always important

Referral and Who Accompanied Patient: Who is the main caretaker, primary physician?

Parent/Guardian Names, Occupations, Daytime Phone numbers:

Chief Complaint: A visit to a nurse or doctor is often for a specific targeted complaint. However, the patient or caregiver will often have other concerns that are only determined through the history taking and discussion. *Use open-ended questions like*, "What brings you in today?" Or, "What can I do for you today?" "Tell me more about that...," often can be used to gather more information while putting the patient as ease by not judging.

History of Present Illness: When did the issue begin, what are the family member's reactions to the illness or concerns, etc.?

Child's Complaint: Is there pain? When did they first feel it? Anything else?

> **NOTE:** The nurse should document whether the complaint is described by the child or the caregiver.

Birth History: Especially for a child under age 2. Where there any complications; was the baby full-term versus premature?

Feeding patterns: When, how often, and what do does the child eat and drink. Were they breastfed? What are the food likes and dislikes? What is the parent's attitude towards the eating choices of the child?

> **NOTE:** The eating and feeding history is the most crucial element of the health history for a child with over-nutrition or under-nutrition concerns. Are the food choices more influenced by the adult or child? This is a chance for the nurse to observe and better understand the patient and their eating attitude, and perhaps understand challenges within their environment – related to eating and nutrition. As nurses, we must take this opportunity to explore the patient and family without judgment. Again, **open-ended questions** work best and allow the patient and caregiver to do the talking and leading, without feeling tested or on-the-spot. *"Tell me about your typical after school snacks,"* versus, *"What do you give John for snack after school?"*

Food Allergies: Include what happens when food is eaten. Some "allergies" are food dislikes or aversions versus a true allergy. Does the child gag or is there itchiness, swelling, difficulty breathing, rash, etc.?

Growth & Development History: How is the child's growth? Perception of growth by the caregiver is crucial to understanding the child's home environment. Cultural differences can play an important role here as the cultural influences of eating can lead to under or overeating by the child. Are there any concerning developmental issues? Any noted growth delay, or cognitive, psychomotor or social issues? Has the child been seen for these concerns? Does the child receive Early Intervention for this and, if so, from what age?

Social Development: How is the child interacting with his or her peers? *"Tell me about his or her friends at home and at school? Do you have any concerns?"*

Sexuality: for children age ten and older, this is an important element of the health history. Is the child curious about gender differences? How is sexuality discussed within the home and at school? What are the child's perceptions? What are the family's cultural attitudes towards sexuality?

Personality: How does the child describe his or her personality? Depending on the age, you might say, *"Tell me three words that describe you."* The parent or guardian should also describe the child's personality. As personality and self-image become more and more intertwined throughout the child's formative and developmental years, this is a crucial element of the psychosocial influences on obesity and wellness.

4: Health History, Review of Systems & Obesity

Now that the patient has set the stage about their overall health history, a **Review of Systems** is taken to ask about each system of the body. This is subjective, as you are asking the patient to describe any medical complaints related to the system. It is not uncommon for a patient to completely skip a major medical issue either due to embarrassment or anxiety in front of a nurse. On the other hand, the review of systems might reveal concerns that were not discovered earlier in the health history. Be patient and understanding. While the review of systems seems largely unrelated to obesity, the health context of the patient must be understood first before you can delve into the issues of concern.

Review of Systems: What are we Asking About?

General: Fatigue, fever/chills, *weight loss* or *gain*, trouble sleeping

Skin: any rashes, lumps, bumps, bruises. During adolescence, the face is a big focus due to social concerns of acne.

Head: Any headaches? If so, further questioning about frequency and type of pain is recommended. Migraines are not uncommon, especially during adolescence, but further assessment is needed. Any lumps, bumps, trauma or injury?

Eyes: Changes in vision, or blurry, or double vision? Does the patient wear contact lenses or glasses? Headaches due to eyestrain are sometimes the first clue to vision change in a child. Date of last eye exam?

Ears: Ear infections, drainage issues, pain, hearing loss, ringing in the ears, hearing aids?

Nose: Congestion, changes in sense of smell, pain, itching, nose bleeds, allergy?

Mouth & Throat: Teeth, gums, soreness, hoarseness, change in quality of the voice, difficulty swallowing, pain swallowing, or ulceration? Date of last dental exam?

Neck: Pain, lumps, bumps, swollen glands, stiffness/difficulty turning or moving?

Respiratory: Breathing trouble – when? Climbing steps versus exercising. Trouble breathing at night? Lung infections, chest pain? Asthma? Wheezing, coughing up blood?

> **NOTE:** With the increase in overweight and obese children and adults, more people are presenting with **sleep apnea** (Muzumdar et,al. 2006). The extra girth of the neck contributes to the breathing issues. Does the patient awaken frequently at night? Are they on CPAP for breathing at night? Have they been evaluated?

Breast: Any lumps, bumps, discharge, pain? Does the patient do self-breast exams?

> **NOTE:** For a developing girl, this topic may be especially sensitive. With the obesity epidemic, we often see that young girls are developing much more rapidly. There has also been lingering controversy regarding hormonal causes of early adolescent development related to additives in foods and chemicals in the environment. While this is beyond our scope, it is important still to understand the patient's perception of their growth.

Genital: As children are becoming sexually active at younger ages, there must be a higher index of suspicion for genital abnormalities than clinicians have assessed in the past.

Female: Painful intercourse, vaginal discharge, itchiness or dryness, abnormal lumps, bumps or pain, STDs?

Male: Painful intercourse, painful erection, erectile dysfunction, abnormal discharge or bleeding, STDs, hernia, masses?

Gastrointestinal: Stomach pain, blood in stool (dark red versus bright red)? Pain when toileting? Constipation, diarrhea (frequency), nausea, vomiting, heartburn, change in appetite

> **NOTE:** This section is exceptionally relevant to obesity and nutrition. More questioning on appetite and changes in weight can be determined here. Again, sensitivity to the patient's insecurities is crucial to obtaining the most accurate review of systems.

Cardiac: chest pain, palpitations, irregular heart rate, trouble breathing, awakening at night?

Musculoskeletal: muscle or joint pain, swelling, redness, stiffness?

> **NOTE:** With increased weight of the child and adult, more people are presenting at younger ages with signs of osteoarthritis. The burden of extra weight on the joints contributes to faster breakdown of cartilage. This will have serious effects on the mobility of even our children.

Vascular: Swelling or cramping in legs, redness, hair loss on legs?

> **NOTE:** As more and more people are now overweight and obese, patients may not notice their leg swelling due to already large extremity size.

Urinary: Frequency, pain, abnormal discharge or bleeding?

Neurologic: Dizziness, fainting, seizures, nausea/vomiting (projectile vomiting), weakness, numbness, tingling, tremor?

Endocrine/Metabolic: Heat or cold intolerance, sweating, frequent urination, excessive thirst, change in appetite?

> **NOTE:** As the rates of obesity steadily climb, so do the rates of Type 2 Diabetes (Savard, M. 2005). Distinguishing changes in appetite related to the pathology of diabetes versus change in appetite due to emotional or environmental factors is important. In the context of overweight individuals, we must have **a high index of suspicion for new onset of Type 2 Diabetes**.

Hematologic: Easy bruising or bleeding?

Psychiatric: Stress, memory loss, depression, nervousness or anxiety?

> **NOTE:** With a focus on obesity and nutrition, there is a likelihood of seeing increased incidence of **eating disorders** as well as patients using various methods of eating as a means to compensate and self treat. Anorexia (absence of appetite) and bulimia (binging and purging) must also be considered in the case of noted changes in appetite and eating patterns, (Rosen, D. 2010).

Though it is beyond the scope of this Guide to diagnose an eating disorder, as nurses, we must be well versed in the many elements of health that interplay to produce such problems.

Summary

In summary, this chapter lays the foundation for taking the health history and assessment of a patient. Nursing care of any patient is about assessment and baseline. Without a proper understanding of the patient's cultural, psychosocial, medical, and physical background, it would be difficult and counterproductive to provide nursing guidance. Nurses must understand the **context** of their patient to know how to best educate and reinforce healthy patterns. Promoting wellness and providing accurate health education relies on individual elements for each patient. The skilled nurse is one who can reach out to the patient through understanding of the individual in the context of their health patterns, whether the patient is morbidly obese, has diabetes or heart disease, or a combination of them all. The nurse must demonstrate knowledge of the human body, the interplay of the systems of the body, and why we nurses must work so hard to promote health and help reduce obesity.

References

Müller, M.J., Asbeck, I., Mast, M., Langnäse, K. and Grund, A. (2001). Prevention of obesity--more than an intention. Concept and first results of the Kiel Obesity Prevention Study. *International Journal of Obesity and Related Metabolic Disorders : Journal of the International Association for the Study of Obesity.* Retrieved 06/10/12 from http://ukpmc.ac.uk/abstract/MED/11466593

Muzumdar, H. & Rao, M. (2006). Pulmonary Dysfunction and Sleep Apnea in Morbid Obesity. *Pediatric Endocrinology* Revised, Supplement 4, 579-83.

Rosen, D. (2010). Identification and Management of Eating Disorders in Children and Adolescents. *Pediatrics Journal by the American Academy of Pediatrics.* Vol. 126 No. 6 December 1, 2010 pp. 1240 -1253 (doi: 10.1542/peds.2010-2821).

Savard, M. (2005). Apples & Pears: the Body Shape Solution for Weight Loss and Wellness. Atria Books, New York.

Van Cauter, E., & Knutson, K.L. (2008). Sleep and the Epidemic of Obesity in Children and Adults. *European Journal of Endocrinology*, 159, Supplement 1, 59-66.

Chapter 5
Obesity, Clinical Findings & Physical Examination

When considering objective health data and factors contributing to a medical/nursing condition, nurses must be able to distinguish between the subjective information (assessed by the patient, nurse, or other provider) versus the clinical data found on exam or by prior report. For instance, a patient might subjectively report, "feeling warm," or the nurse might indicate that a patient is febrile. In both instances, these descriptions are subjective. To clinically determine a fever, the numeric temperature (such as 101.8°F) is objective and clinical. Without defining measureable clinical characteristics, there would be little way to monitor improvement or change, or determine how quickly or assertively to implement a plan. Similarly, to establish whether or not a patient is clinically obese or overweight and devise a plan, nurses must have certain measureable data and information by which to understand the problem.

When nurses care for an overweight, obese, or at risk patient, many questions must be answered. In the previous chapter, we learned how to gather a Health History and Review of Systems to have the patient help answer the "Who, What, When, Where, Why, and How" questions. Now, the nurse must answer the questions through thorough collection of data and clinical examination. Nurses gather objective data via use of measurement tools and data, conducting a physical examination, and documenting the results thoroughly.

At a minimum, a nurse must gather the following:
- Name, Age, and Gender
- Height, Weight, BMI
- Health habits: Smoker, Alcohol consumption, illicit drugs, herbal/vitamins
- Medications: prescription, over the counter (OTC), and herbal remedies
- Blood Pressure, pulse, respirations
- Blood sugar, lipid panel, metabolic panel, thyroid, etc.
- History of illnesses: diabetes, heart disease, joint disease, hypertension, etc.
- Physical Exam: with focus on heart, lungs, abdomen, skin, extremities, etc.

Despite the objective nature of the physical exam and clinical findings, nurses and their patients must understand the dynamic nature and variability of objective measurements. Nurses must be able to recognize normal variability from a patient's baseline as compared to what might be a significant or atypical change. Assessing changes in a patient's clinical data (as they relate to their baseline) is necessary to monitor for the efficacy of interventions, and to further develop appropriate nursing care plans. Whether the measurement is weight, blood pressure, cholesterol, or blood sugar, these clinical measurements can have some degree of change without identifying a problem, per se. Still, clinical measurements and clinical definitions are essential to help establish a problem, monitor the problem, and assess improvement or change in status. Nurses must remember that without proper and thorough documentation to relay the facts and demonstrate trends in the objective information, the gathered information is useless. Therefore, progress notes are a systematic and chronological look at the problem to help build a picture of what is happening, what should happen, and what has happened.

> Chapter 5 Objectives:
> 1. Appraise if a patient is obese versus overweight
> 2. Chart the use of measurements: height, weight, and BMI
> 3. Discuss the purpose of monitoring growth using growth charts
> 4. Infer physical exam findings in an overweight or obese patient

In a medical sense, obesity is defined according to a formula or ratio of a person's weight compared to his or her height. This calculation of *Body Mass Index* (BMI) has been determined to be a relatively consistent measurement for obesity. However, it must be noted that the BMI is still relative not only to the patient's weight and height, but also to the general population's weight and height. That means for the *average* person, BMI can be a fairly accurate measurement of body fat. BMI provides a numerical range to determine if a person is overweight, underweight, or obese based on a series of parameters. Note that while BMI is the current "gold standard" of measurement for defining obesity, it is not necessarily the most specific measurement. Since BMI is inexpensive and easy to measure, it can be widely used as a screening tool.

Remember that, as with any screening tool, there are certain situations in which the measurement is not sensitive and can provide false results. For instance, in the case of an athlete or someone with a very different body build, the BMI might be inaccurate and *overestimate* the person's relative body fat. A well-toned athlete can have essentially no body fat, yet have a high BMI due to the weight to height ratio (because muscle is heavier than fat).

Table 5-1. Standard BMI and Weight Status

BMI	Weight Status
Below 18.5	Underweight
18.5 – 24.9	Normal
25.0 – 29.9	Overweight
30.0 and Above	Obese

Reprinted with permission from CDC.gov.

While a BMI over 25 (see chart) is considered overweight, there are other accepted measurements used, as well, to determine whether a person is overweight or obese. (For example, skin fold measurements had been used widely, but have now been replaced by BMI.) Also, simple formulas for a person's appropriate weight have been used as a guide, though without proven efficacy.

I, Debbie, remember using the following formula:

100 lbs + ((# of inches over 5ft.) x 5lbs) = Average weight of woman
110 + ((# inches over 5ft.) x 5 lbs) = Average weight of man

This calculation, though an appropriate approximation for adults, is more an estimate of weight than a calculation of body mass. A nurse can just as easily assess a high or low body weight by visual assessment (though this chapter focuses on objective data). Do not underestimate your training as a healthcare professional. Measurements are a guide, but you must use your education and instincts. If you can visually see an increase in weight or see a family trend of obesity, do not refrain from mentioning your concerns, especially if you are not in the appropriate setting to take actual measurements. Prevention is paramount.

How is BMI Calculated?

As the Centers for Disease Control and Prevention is the accepted standard for health guidelines in the United States, let us look at their exact guidelines and then try to decipher what they mean.

Adult BMI is calculated as follows:

English BMI Formula
BMI= (Weight in Pounds/(Height in Inches)^2) x 703

Metric BMI Formula
BMI= Weight in Kilograms/(Height in Meters)^2

5: Obesity, Clinical Findings & Physical Examination

The previous calculation seems daunting, so a simpler height chart can be used to find BMIs that correspond to a specific height. For the height of 5' 9", the table below gives the corresponding BMI ranges and the weight status categories for this sample height:

Table 5-2 Weight Range/Status and BMI for 5' 9" Sample Height

Height	Weight Range	BMI	Weight Status
5' 9"	124 lbs or less	Below 18.5	Underweight
	125 lbs to 168 lbs	18.5 to 24.9	Normal
	169 lbs to 202 lbs	25.0 to 29.9	Overweight
	203 lbs or more	30 or higher	Obese

Reprinted with permission from CDC.gov.

BMI for Children

All nurses remember the need to calculate medication dosages for children during their pediatric clinical rotations. Pediatric nurses taught us to weigh diapers to assess output, measure milk consumption from a bottle, and calculate intravenous drip rates for babies and infants. Since we learn how weight affects nursing care of children, the use of different parameters for children is clear. Simiarly, the proper use of measurement tools, including growth charts for different ages and gender are needed. Until the past decade, measuring BMI for children was not a high priority. Nurses and clinicians did not always routinely measure BMI and mostly opted for simple height and weight measurements along a curve. But with the increase of childhood obesity over the past twenty years, there has been a greater focus on accurate measurements to monitor trends in growth, which is why the BMI is now being used more regularly by clinicians.

While BMI appears to be the best measurement we have right now, there remains controversy regarding its use. With the childhood obesity epidemic, there has been much research on the success of routine BMI measurements in school settings to look for at-risk populations with increased BMI. However, there remains a question of the benefit versus the cost of routine BMI measurements. Some states are now adopting legislation that requires routine BMI measurements, but there remains a big issue – what next? This policy can show data, but lacks the ability to help implement the support and education needed to reverse the trend toward high BMI and obesity among children.

While a child's BMI is calculated the same way, children under the age of 20 are age- and gender-specific for a more accurate measurement. *Chapter 7 will delve into the complexities of child development and monitoring the many gender- and age-specific growth charts.* There are so many charts, graphs, formulas, and measurements to determine obesity that even a trained scientist or mathematician can get dizzy. To simplify our understanding, two graphs for childhood obesity BMI measurements are included to understand how height and weight is used to monitor growth along a curve. Note that there is a separate CDC graph for boys and girls ages 2 to 20 years. *It is essential to understand that boys and girls are different and grow along different trajectories.* (*See Figures 5-1, 2: Growth Charts*, on the following pages).

The limitations of growth charts and BMI use as diagnostic tools for obesity must be understood. Growth charts are a *tool* using BMI as a *measurement* to help provide concrete numbers to follow growth patterns. They are useful to compare children and young adults to their own prior measurements, and to measurements of a typical child of that age, nothing more.

Let us compare the use of BMI for someone who is overweight to the temperature of someone who is sick. If we take a person's temperature and determine that the patient has a fever (ie. 101.4 F), the medical staff will diagnose, treat, and care for the patient. For example, if the fever corresponds to an ear infection, antibiotics may be given, but the fever is still treated empirically with Acetominophen and fluids. Similarly, if a BMI is taken and determined to be high, there must be a *plan*. How will the patient be educated about their high BMI? And how relevant is the BMI to that individual person?

This is why BMI in the absence of a health history and physical exam would make a health management plan incomplete and difficult to carry out. Remember that for certain people (athletes, for example), a high BMI is *not* indicative of obesity. Therefore, the entire physical exam must be considered. The following discussion of physical exams gives helpful notes to understand what to look for on physical exam, and what clinical observations a nurse might make in the context of an overweight or obese patient.

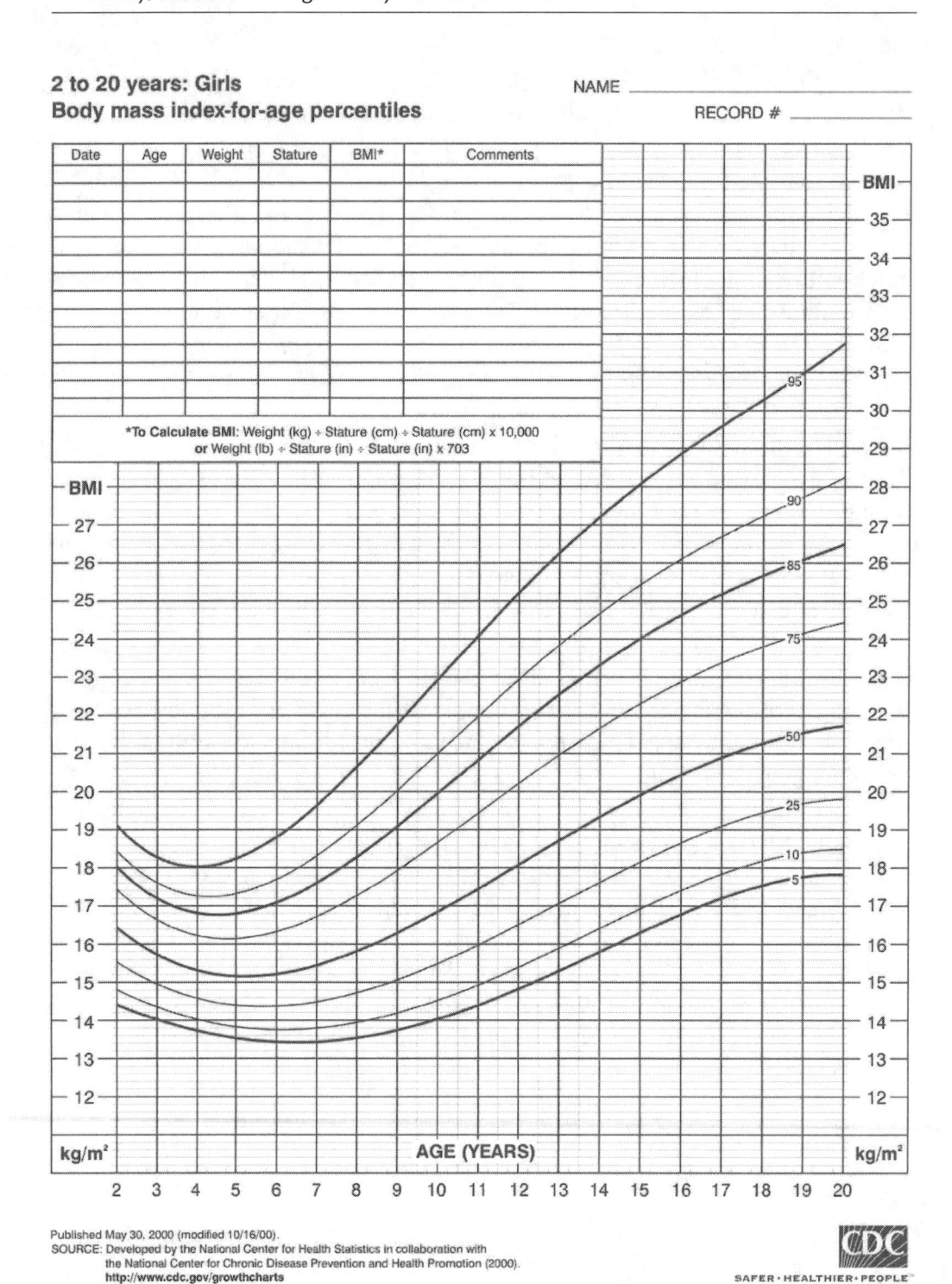

5: Obesity, Clinical Findings & Physical Examination

Figure 5-1. Girls, Body Mass Index-For-Age Percentiles (2–20 Years)
Reprinted with permission from the Center for Disease Control and Prevention.
Chart has not been modified from original form.

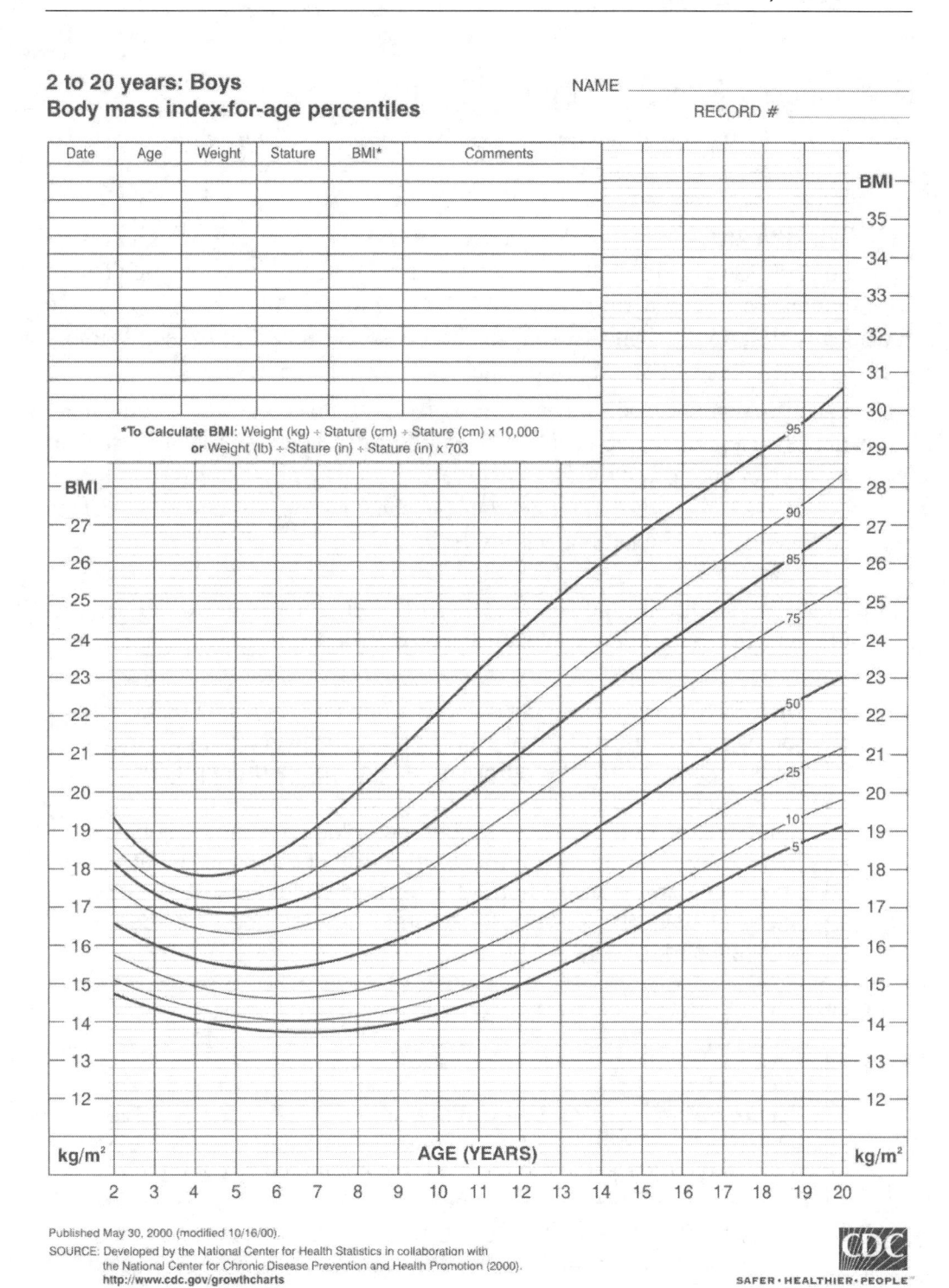

Figure 5-2. Boys, Body Mass Index-For-Age Percentiles (2–20 Years)
Reprinted with permission from the Center for Disease Control and Prevention.
Chart has not been modified from original form.

How Obesity Affects a Physical Exam

*** A "normal" exam is listed, with **NOTES** to indicate abnormalities that may be found related to obesity.*

GENERAL APPEARANCE: "Well developed, well nourished" was always a nursing descriptive phrase to indicate the patient is not malnourished or cachectic. Today, with so many overweight and obese adults, it becomes all the more important to specifically describe patients as overweight, obese, or morbidly obese. Without taking a BMI, this is admittedly only subjective and descriptive.

A nurse or doctor looking back through prior notes will want to understand the patient's baseline. If the baseline from 2009 describes a patient as slender with ill-fitting clothing, and the 2012 general appearance now describes the same patient as overweight, this can guide your physical assessment and exam. (One question to ask: Does the patient acknowledge a weight gain?)

HEAD: normocephalic (normal shape and size). Remember that for babies it is crucial for a head circumference to be measured as part of the growth parameters.

> **NOTE:** While obesity can cause additional facial adiposity, the cranium remains of normal size. Babies or adults with abnormally large heads could be showing a sign of hydrocephalus (or macrocephaly from other causes, or in more acute cases, from internal bleeding) and may require neurological examination and ultrasound, CT or MRI. There are certainly genetic variations in cranial size that are normal, yet there should also be a high index of suspicion for abnormally small or large head size due to skeletal abnormalities.

EYES: PERRL, EOMI. Vision grossly intact.

> **NOTE:** Typically, a nurse will not do a full fundoscopic exam. Neurological eye exams are more commonly conducted to test eye movements, as part of a neuro assessment for in-patient neurology patients.

> **ADDITIONAL NOTE:** Since obese patients are at higher risk of diabetes, hypertension, and hypercholesterolemia, assessing the eyes for indication of diabetic retinopathy, arcus senilus, and glaucoma are all necessary. Interestingly, a study from the Netherlands found that increased BMI in women, while increasing eye pressure, reduced the risk of glaucoma. (Ramdas, Archives of Ophthalmology, May 2011).

EARS: External auditory canals and TMs clear, hearing grossly intact. (The ears should not be affected by obesity.)

NOSE: No nasal discharge. (The nose should not be affected by obesity.)

THROAT: Oral cavity and pharynx normal. No inflammation, swelling, exudate, or lesions. Teeth and gingiva in good general condition.

> *NOTE:* The throat should not be affected directly by obesity, yet obesity significantly increases the risk of upper airway obstruction and sleep apnea. Therefore, inspect the tonsils and adenoids carefully, but also pay attention to neck girth and other signs of obesity. BMI must be considered. 70% of people with BMI of 40 or greater have obstructive sleep apnea (Ludman et al, 2007).

CARDIAC: Normal S1 and S2. No S3, S4 or murmurs. Rate and rhythm are regular. There is no peripheral edema, cyanosis or pallor. Extremities are warm. Capillary refill <2 seconds. No bruits.

> *NOTE:* A cardiac exam is essential for an overweight or obese patient because the risk of heart disease is increased, as is the risk of hypertension and hypercholesterolemia. The larger the person, the more demand there is on the heart to perfuse the entire body. (When women are pregnant, there is 70% more blood perfusing through the body to compensate for the added work of nurturing the fetus. The body is regulated to do this.) In an overweight body, the heart may struggle to keep up with the added demands. Listen very carefully for an irregular heart beat and/or murmurs and feel pulses, as these are all crucial. Feeling pulses on an obese person may be more difficult. Sometimes, a Doppler will be needed to listen for pedal pulses.

> *ADDITIONAL NOTE:* Landmarks for an accurate and successful heart exam are more difficult to find on an overweight or obese patient. Take the time to reposition the patient as needed to accurately auscultate and palpate for heart sounds and pulses.

LUNGS: Clear to auscultation (CTA) and percussion without rales, rhonchi, wheezing or diminished breath sounds.

> *NOTE:* Wheezing or coughing can be misunderstood to be pulmonary in nature, when, really, they can be related to the heart and obesity. In the context of an obese patient, it is crucial to distinguish between abnormal pulmonary exam and abnormal

(Continued)

> cardiac exam. The treatment would be very different. More evidence over the past decade shows links between pulmonary and respiratory conditions and obesity. Sleep apnea, asthma, and respiratory capacity related to exercise are related to obesity (Muzudmar, 2006).

MUSCULOSKELETAL: Adequately aligned spine. ROM intact spine and extremities. No joint erythema or tenderness. Normal muscular development. Normal gait.

> ***NOTE:*** Obese patients are at risk of joint disease due to the added weight and stress on joints. (It is not uncommon to see younger patients with musculoskeletal complaints than ever before.) Osteoarthritis from excessive weight can severely limit ROM. But be sure that your exam assesses whether the limited ROM is due to the musculoskeletal system versus the obesity of the patient. Limited ROM does not necessarily signify joint conditions. (Questions to consider: *Is there pain? Swelling? Warmth? Redness?*)

NECK: Neck supple, non-tender without lymphadenopathy, masses or thyromegaly.

BACK: Normal gait and posture, no spinal deformity, symmetry of spinal muscles, without tenderness, decreased ROM or spasm.

> ***NOTE:*** Obesity and added weight have contributed to a higher risk of chronic back pain. Careful examination of ROM and gait are crucial. Follow-up questions might be warranted to assess more history of the pain. To what does the patient attribute his or her back pain?

EXTREMITIES: No joint abnormality. No edema. Peripheral pulses intact. No varicosities.

LOWER EXTREMITY: Examination of both feet reveals all toes to be normal in size and symmetry, normal range of motion, normal sensation with distal capillary filling of less than 2 seconds without tenderness, swelling, discoloration, nodules, weakness or deformity; examination of both ankles, knees, legs, and hips reveals normal range of motion, normal sensation without tenderness, swelling, discoloration, crepitus, weakness or deformity.

> **NOTE:** Assessing whether lower extremity swelling is due to fluid or subcutaneous fat can be very tricky. If there is pitting edema, you can more clearly ascertain that there is fluid retention. Non-pitting edema versus extra subcutneous fat requires more skill to determine. The patient's baseline is crucial here. Further questioning related to pain, soreness, and the need to elevate may be required. The patient's cardiac history and exam needs to be reviewed, as well, to determine if the edema is related to venous stasis, heart failure, or potential blood clot (DVT). The nurse must have a high index of suspicion, since obesity can mask a true medical need for extremity edema evaluation.

NEUROLOGICAL: CN II-XII intact. Strength and sensation symmetric and intact. Reflexes 2+ throughout. Cerebellar testing normal.

> **NOTE:** Landmarks for reflexes are more difficult due to increased size of the patient. Be patient and make sure you hit the target spot before assessing reflexes to be normal.

SKIN: Skin normal color, texture and turgor with no lesions or bruises.

> **NOTE:** Due to increased skin surface area on obese patients, nurses must take the time to examine the skin thoroughly. *Skin folds* must be examined, as well, to look for rashes, fungal infections, and yeast infections. (The breasts should be lifted gently to look for moisture or rashes, as should abdominal folds.) Explaining to the patient what your exam is looking for (rashes, redness) can save some embarrassment on the part of the patient, who already feels vulnerable during a thorough skin exam.
>
> Chafing between the legs, sometimes appearing as a more sinister diagnosis, can simply be from rubbing and chafing of the legs when the patient walks. Encourage the patient to use barrier creams and wear comfortable pants (rather than shorts) to help protect against friction while walking.

PSYCHIATRIC: The mental examination revealed the patient was oriented to person, place, and time. The patient was able to demonstrate good judgement and reason, without hallucinations, abnormal affect or abnormal behaviors during the examination. Patient is not suicidal.

5: Obesity, Clinical Findings & Physical Examination

> **NOTE:** Because the psychiatric status of the patient can largely influence eating patterns, assessing for depression, anxiety, and other psychiatric symptoms is important. Further studies, such as a the *Geriatric Depression Scale* for older adults, should be included in the assessment, if applicable.

In nursing school, many nurses practiced physical examination on their nursing peers, and thus did not always have the opportunity to discover abnormal findings. However, even becoming well versed in a typical, healthy or normal physical exam can provide the needed experience to translate into the skills needed when nurses do discover a problem. Because nurses learn a thorough and stepwise method of conducting even a normal exam, they can understand what findings they should not see, regardless of whether they are trained well enough to diagnose the exact problem. For instance, when I, Debbie, had a nurse practitioner student conduct a physical exam on me during my course of study, she discovered a heart murmur. She certainly did not know the type of murmur (benign or not), but understood that the heart sounds were not within the "normal" that she was trained to hear. By telling me about the possible murmur, I could then refer myself to physician who could further assess and diagnose. After a visit to the doctor, an echocardiogram, and a question of mitral valve regurgitation, the murmur was deemed benign. If the echocardiogram were to have indicated mitral valve prolapse, I would pursue prophylactic antibiotics before dental procedures (to prevent infection of the heart from bacteria into the bloodstream).

We explain the above anecdotal story so that nurses can understand:
- *WHY* we conduct a thorough exam
- *WHY* we must explain and document our results
- *WHY* we learn what findings are normal or abnormal in relationship to obesity and chronic conditions
- *HOW* it affects our further management, interventions, and goals

Obesity is a measurable, identifiable, and clinical condition that must be assessed and monitored. Because there has been little medical and nursing focus on generalized obesity, unless in the context of pre-existing medical conditions, it will take time for healthcare providers to adopt obesity as a condition we must fully address within the scope of physical examination. Nurses must become well versed in findings related to obesity that can contribute to other health conditions. Knowing the importance of a full heart, lung, abdominal, musculoskeletal, and skin exam is crucial to help set goals and interventions for obese, overweight, or at risk individuals.

References

Centers for Disease Control and Prevention. CDC 24/7: Saving Lives. Protecting People. Retrieved 02/15/12 from http://www.cdc.gov/healthyweight/assessing/bmi/adult_bmi/index.html

Centers for Disease Control and Prevention. CDC 24/7: Saving Lives. Protecting People. Retrieved 06/06/12 from http://www.cdc.gov/growthcharts

Ludman, H., & Bradley, P.J. (2007). *ABC of Ear, Nose and Throat*. Oxford: Blackwell Publishing.

Muzumdar, H., & Rao, M., (2006). Pulmonary Dysfunction and Sleep Apnea in Morbid Obesity. *Pediatric Endocrinology* Revised, Supplement 4, 579-83.

Ramdas, W.D., Van Koolwijk, L.M., Lemij, H.G., Pasutto, F., Cree, A.J., and Thorleifsson, G. (2011) Common genetic variants associated with open-angle glaucoma. *Human Molecular Genetics*, Archives of Ophthalmology, retrieved 05/07/12 from http://www.ncbi.nlm.nih.gov/pubmed/21427129?dopt=Abstract

Chapter 6
Underlying Disability & Obesity

In 2010, the prevalence of non-institutionalized disabled males and females of all ages, races, and ethnicities was 11.9% of the United States population (Erickson et. al, 2012). Having a hearing, visual, ambulatory, cognitive, self-care, or independent living disability were the six criteria that identified and defined a "disability." Although this survey of over 3 million people was based on a U.S. Census Bureau calculation from 2008, it is not possible to determine the exact nature and degree of disability within this sample population. However, in this chapter, we highlight the relatively high prevalence of people with disabilities (over 33 million people in America have at least one disability, as per the above survey), and the need to identify, understand, and assess the unique needs of people with disabilities, whether the patients are young or older.

In this chapter, we explore how *already* having a disability can *predispose* an individual to become obese. The prevalence of obesity among individuals with disabilities is generally not due to a genetic predisposition towards obesity, per se, but rather due to impaired access or reduced ability to lead a healthy lifestyle. The diagnosis of a disability can be a relatively objective and identifiable characteristic of the patient. Although certain components of a disability are subjective, like the extent to which an individual is impaired, the nurse must consider how the disability can or will affect the patient's care plan, mobility, and/or communicative ability. We must not ignore the significant way in which disability, compounded with obesity, can increase health risk and make healthy living an even greater challenge.

> Chapter 6 Objectives:
> 1. Determine the impact of underlying disability on obesity
> 2. Explain nutritional and physical limitations of individuals with disabilities
> 3. Express how to advocate for children and adults with disabilities

While the prevalence of childhood obesity has doubled in the United States, the prevalence of obesity for disabled children is TWICE as high as among children without disabilities (Reinehr et al, 2010). This is an incredibly large number, making the obesity issue even more significant for this population of children already faced with significant health and medical needs. For this reason, we dedicate a chapter to understanding obesity in the context of children with disabilities (and, of course, these children often become adults with disabilities). Awareness, prevention, and education are critical, and must be considered earlier rather than later.

Research shows that, already by the age of three, marked differences in prevalence of overweight and obese disabled children compared to their counterparts can be found (Reinehr et al., 2010). Unfortunately, even in the case of certain disabilities, the diagnoses are not made until later, once health patterns and weight issues have begun. Helping patients, families, and providers understand the significance of obesity among ALL children is a critical first, so that, even in the face of disability, parents can be well equipped and educated on the need for healthy behaviors.

Many of us are aware of the increase in medical and developmental diagnoses among children these days. It seems that a new condition with a new treatment is discussed almost daily. Regardless of the reasons for this, we will now see more and more children with disabilities, and thus must understand how to best encourage the same nutrition and fitness needs to reduce obesity for them, as we would for others.

Numerous congenital medical and developmental conditions can have a tremendous effect on the health, nutritional status, and activity ability of children with disabilities. We commonly hear about children with developmental conditions like autism, Asperger's, Attention Deficit Hyperactivity Disorder, etc., and most people do not quite understand how this might affect their health needs beyond effective communication. Research has found that children with developmental delays are more likely to spend more time in front of the television, and we already know this increases the risk of obesity. What might seem a "subtle" disability must be considered from many perspectives. The various disabilities among children, and the extent to which these disabilities affect our children's healthy living, challenges all of us to understand each child uniquely in so many ways: medically, educationally, and emotionally.

Due to the chronic nature of childhood disability, and sometimes the lack of or access to needed services, conditions such as autism, cerebral palsy, spina bifida, Down's syndrome, asthma, deafness, and blindness can increase the risk of children with these conditions becoming overweight or obese. Compared to their healthy counterparts, U.S. children and adolescents with limited functional mobility showed rates of 30% obesity (among disabled) versus 16% (among healthy), and for children with a learning disability, the rate of 21.9% obesity (disabled) compared to 15.7% (among healthy) (Reinehr et al, 2010).

These differences are significant and must highlight the need for special consideration and awareness of obesity issues among children with many types of conditions, both physical and cognitive in nature. One in 33 infants is born with a birth defect (CDC, 2012).

Let us not forget that many children with disabilities already have higher risk factors for heart disease, impaired nutrition, immobility, and more. Epidemiologists (along with healthcare providers) agree that the obesity epidemic will increase the incidence of many chronic conditions including heart disease, joint problems, liver issues, sleep apnea, asthma, and more. All of these conditions will likely present at earlier and earlier ages influenced by obesity, and will lead to more people with long-term disabilities. Prevention is key, and children are the priority.

> The HERO Program promotes health education and fitness programming for children of all levels and medical conditions. Thus far, we have worked with children with autism and spina bifida, for which a child requires urinary catheterization. Whether or not the child required extra adult supervision, or a break for catheterization, accommodation is always a priority. As is health education for ALL children, regardless of ability or disability, obese or not. We must encourage caregivers and teachers to understand that, just as early intervention for occupational therapy or speech therapy is needed, likewise health education could be implemented to focus on the need for proper nutrition and fitness.

As we emphasize throughout this book, people challenged by obesity are faced with many social and health challenges. Now consider those who have concomitant physical and/or developmental challenges, which further compound an already complex health issue. These individuals must now rely on caregivers not only for daily living and medical needs, but also for extra intervention and assistance to enhance nutrition and physical activity needs to prevent or reduce obesity (Doody et al 2012).

How many Americans have disabilities? According to the 2008 U.S. Census Bureau Survey, 54.4 million Americans have disabilities (Brault, 2008). This is 19% of the non-institutionalized population (and remember, this is the *reported* population).

Below is a breakdown of the disabled population by age:
- **5 percent** of children ages 5 to 17 have disabilities.
- **10 percent** of people ages 18 to 64 have disabilities.
- **38 percent** of adults ages 65 and older have disabilities.

With further breakdown by age, we see that the prevalence of disability among children under age 15 rises dramatically and exponentially:

- **Under age 3**, 1.8% have disabilities
- **Age 3 to age 5**, 3.6% have disabilities
- **Age 6 to age 14**, 12.4% have disabilities

(United States Census Bureau 2005.)

Many causes may explain the increase in the percentage of disability among children, including certain conditions, which manifest at a later age, school assistance in diagnosing a disability and, as children age and school expectations increase, children's limitations (whether academic, physical, or psychosocial) become more pronounced. Thus, the older a child gets without making expected cognitive or physical progress can make an underlying disability become more apparent.

Not all disabilities are created equal. For example, the U.S. Census Bureau distinguishes between developmental delays and difficulty in walking or running when it comes to younger children. Once children reach school age, the Census Bureau further defines disability in children according to educational and learning disabilities (as well as physical disabilities). The majority of disabilities tend to fall under the umbrella of speech and language disabilities, so not all conditions affect our main focus of wellness and nutrition; that said, there are still a significant number of children with other types of disabilities who *do* need our help. We must not ignore this vital section of the population.

For this chapter, we will define individuals with disabilities as those with physical or cognitive limitations for whom daily life is altered. Understanding that some individuals have only physical disability, only cognitive disability, or both, nurses must recognize how *all* impairments can limit a child's capacity to access health care and initiate healthy behaviors.

In nursing school, there is little focus on *disability* aside from acute illness-induced disability or chronic illness. That is, we learn how to care for the post-surgical patient when we learn to toilet, bathe, and help them ambulate. But other than experiencing a brief community health rotation, we may have learned little about how the chronically disabled individual leads his daily life outside of our care. We also may have learned the names of certain more common genetic disorders such as trisomy 21, cerebral palsy, or muscular dystrophy. But, globally and grossly, we may not have learned the "big picture" of disability, and many of us certainly were not fully exposed to the range and severity of disabilities in real life. In fact, even after completing nursing school and during real practice, we still may not have been exposed to the realities of people who live with disabilities.

In today's society, with children and adults who are not already challenged, the ability or inclination to pursue activity and fitness is already severely diminished. Even children with no prior health history to limit their abilities are less likely to maintain an active and nutritionally balanced lifestyle today than twenty years ago. The real question is, if these numbers are so extreme for the *typical* population of children, how are disabled children affected? Researchers (Reinehr et al., 2010) reviewed 38 publications related to obesity and children with disabilities, and there remains a consistent and significant association between obesity and children with disabilities. In a nutshell, disability compounds the already evident challenges that our children face in a world of high tech, fast-paced, yet highly sedentary lifestyles.

How can our population of children and adults with prior disabilities improve their health behaviors? They cannot do this alone; as previously stated, many are reliant upon their caregivers. And their caregiver might be *you*, the *nurse* – or the caregivers are reliant on *you*, the *nurse*.

Fortunately, there are federal and state programs in place to provide necessary services for children from birth to age 2 with special needs. *Early intervention* is the general term for these ancillary medical/educational services that include speech therapy, occupational therapy, vision-impaired and hearing-impaired instruction, etc.

According to the Healthy People 2020 data, 91% of children with disabilities (birth-2 years) received early intervention services in community-based or home settings in 2007. Because such a high percentage of children received these services (and the Healthy People 2020 goal is to increase the percentage to 95%), it would seem natural that health education and wellness for a child with disabilities could be introduced to the parents at this stage. Or, at a minimum, provide a resource guide for parents to maintain for future needs (HHS, 2012).

Beyond the age of early intervention, services for children with special needs become more fragmented. Pediatricians and medical facilities provide certain services, the schools provide other services, but, unfortunately, there is little communication between the two. As disabled children continue through school, there is such a wide variation by city, state, county, hospital, and support network, etc., that the likelihood of a child falling through the cracks of society is enormous.

> **NOTE:** For school-aged children with disabilities, the best resource is another parent who has navigated the same system. Finding a network of other parents, whether in person or on the Web, can provide the parents with a channel or forum for troubleshooting their barriers in school and out. For example, a pro-active parent or caregiver will sometimes rally other parents to send their children to typical extracurricular activities, despite their limited abilities.

With the Individuals with Disabilities Education Act of 2004 (the most recent version), there are provisions to ensure that children with disabilities receive a "Free and Pubic Education" (FAPE). Becoming familiar with the rules can help the parent advocate for their child. As this guide focuses on wellness to reduce obesity, and with the full knowledge that children with disabilities are *already* challenged, knowing the child's rights to participate in school programming is essential.

From IDEA.ED.GOV (US Department of Education):
> Section 300.107(a), regarding nonacademic services, has been revised to specify the steps each public agency must take, including the provision of supplementary aids and services determined appropriate and necessary by the child's IEP Team, to provide nonacademic and extracurricular services and activities in the manner necessary to afford children with disabilities an equal opportunity for participation in those services and activities.
>
> Proposed Sec. 300.108(a), regarding physical education services, has been revised to specify that **physical education must be made available to all children with disabilities receiving FAPE, unless the public agency enrolls children without disabilities and does not provide physical education to children without disabilities in the same grades.**

This means that if other children have weekly P.E., so shall the child with disabilities, and they (the public agencies, including public schools) need to accommodate the child to enable him/her to participate. In theory, if the child needs a wheelchair only for P.E. to be able to go out on the field, then they should provide one for that specific use. Leaving a child to sit on a bench while peers are at P.E. is not acceptable and should be argued.

Part of the problem is that physical education teachers may not have taught a child with disabilities before, much less a child with a specific type of disability. This means those teachers may take the easy option of allowing the disabled child to sit out of physical activity. But this is not acceptable, because it is *imperative* for children with disabilities to engage in whatever suitable components of physical activity they can. So in the case of the reluctant P.E. teacher, whomever advocates for the child in question needs to highlight what the disabled child still can *do*, rather than what he or she cannot.

Most exercises can be *adjusted* in some form to *accommodate* a range of disabilities, which is why, with a little work, most P.E. teachers should be willing to help any child (with or without a disability) become more active. After all, P.E. teachers, by nature, should want all children to attain whatever level of fitness they can; if you couch your arguments in just that way, it may help the P.E. teacher understand you.

If the child in question requires constant supervision, do not let this be an obstacle! **Advocate for these children** – they have just as many rights as anyone else. And they certainly need to be just as active – if not more so – than their counterparts.

For a physically disabled child or adult, *mobility* is the greatest challenge to an active lifestyle. How can we encourage fitness and adapt fitness requirements and activities for individuals bound to a bed, walker, or wheelchair? Does our patient have the resources and adaptive mobility devices they need? Getting the right device (cane, walker, wheelchair, etc.) can be an uphill battle at best. In a school setting, many mobility devices can be requested for school use (and often at *no cost*, as this is part of maintaining the *"least restrictive environment"* for the child). While wheelchairs may not be eligible for these free programs, depending on the state or municipality in which you live, there might still be ways to obtain devices through advocacy programs and nonprofit organizations.

Remember that helping any individual with disabilities, especially a child, requires a multidisciplinary approach. In the case of a disabled child, hard work on the part of the parents, child, nursing/medical/therapy team, and early intervention program is vital to a successful outcome for that child. The greatest tragedy for an already physically challenged child is for the people around him or her to give up before the child has a chance to understand, accept and compensate for physical limitations.

It is crucial that you help the disabled child find the right path to success. And you, as the nurse, having seen more children with disabilities than the average citizen, are in a vital position to pass this message along. Children, even with tremendous disabilities (blindness, musculoskeletal, neurological, or more), can overcome more than some scientific, medically-driven nurses will believe. Be sure to look at the individual child in question, and ask yourself: what can I do to help this person/this family? How can I help advocate for this child?

Your assistance as a nurse will be very helpful, because, mostly, parents need some hope, or maybe a focus that is not directly linked to their child's disability. This is not to say that we should tell parents of children with paraplegia that those children will wake up in a few months and walk again. But, sometimes, offering a parent a bit of guidance as to what type of interventions may be available (in order to help the child) can be useful.

As the nurse, you can effectively encourage a parent or caregiver to continue helping the disabled child or adult to exercise, even via passive ROM exercises. Without exercise, muscles will atrophy. After a debilitating stroke (whether a pediatric or adult stroke patient), a patient without active and passive range of motion exercises will likely have contractures of the unused extremities. We also know that this same patient, who is bedridden and has a lower metabolic rate, does not have the same caloric requirements as an active person of the same age, weight, and height.

Encouraging parents to channel their desire to improve the health of their child can encompass even small changes in the child's eating and activity levels. But remember that the parent of a disabled child is often overwhelmed, may not know where to begin, and might have difficulty prioritizing how to best support the needs of the medically or physically challenged child. This is why talking about small, doable changes is probably the very best thing you can do in the short term to help the parents of a newly disabled (or newly-diagnosed) child.

If a child struggles to breathe, and the parent's focus is (for obvious reasons) on the child's airway, improving the child's eating is not the primary concern. But, because of the many scary and extremely challenging needs of disabled children, the cycle of disability and obesity can perpetuate, especially as more gaps in medical care ensue. This is why nutritional help must be offered, even if parents (or children) don't seem to see the need for it.

The transition between child and adult in the face of disability is complicated by fragmented care and the confusion regarding where to turn in order to find good and meaningful help. According to Healthy People 2020, only 41.2 % of youths with special needs had medical providers discuss transition planning from pediatric to adult health care in 2005 to 2006. Without this transitional planning, and with the complex healthcare needs of a young adult with special needs, the barriers to care increase, the needs of the patient also increase, and access to health care and health promotion activities will eventually be decreased. This is why such transitional planning is absolutely essential, lest a disabled young adult fall right through the cracks.

Another goal of Healthy People 2020 is to reduce the barriers to health and wellness programs for people with disabilities, yet there is no current data to explore how significant the barriers truly are. While there are federal laws to help protect and accommodate people with disabilities, in reality, there remain many gaps for an already challenged individual. (HHS, 2012). To help tackle these gaps in healthcare for the physically impaired child or adult, we must ask a few questions:

What are the physical limitations?
- Can the child use his or her upper body?
- Can the child use his or her lower body?
- Does he/she have coordinated movements?
- What activities would be realistic for the child to pursue?
- What activities could possibly help improve his or her condition?

Understanding the child's physical condition and his or her physical and social environment is needed in order to best explore options for physical activity for the child. Sometimes, thinking "outside the box" is necessary. A team approach and a willingness to try new activities should be encouraged.

Here's a personal example from Debbie:

***

DEBBIE'S STORY: When my daughter was one month old, I was told that she would not develop "on target" with other children due to a bone condition. At the time, I anticipated delayed crawling and walking, and gait instability.

She was evaluated by a physical therapist at age 10 weeks. At this time, I was told she would have difficulty sitting up and walking. This prognosis turned out to be accurate. Wanting to give my daughter the greatest opportunity for success, I made sure that she began physical therapy before age one.

I soon learned she also was progressively losing her vision. This meant her mobility had additional challenges. Therapists worked on using many variations of push toys to help her walk, and to graduate her into use of a mobility white-tipped cane for the blind.

What should have been a typical milestone of walking and navigating her environment took a tremendous twist. Blind and physically impaired, physical activity took more effort for her, requiring special therapists who helped to increase her opportunities to interact in her physical environment.

A proactive early intervention teacher encouraged my daughter to pursue hippo therapy (the use of horseback riding as a therapeutic way to improve trunk stability). I was told that because horses walk on four legs, the natural forward *and* sideways gait of the horse helps to strengthen the rider's torso. Though it seemed ridiculous to pursue horseback riding for an eighteen-month-old disabled child, I now attribute some of her perseverance and endurance to this early therapy. And lo and behold, it was paid for by the state through early intervention, as we demonstrated a need for it.

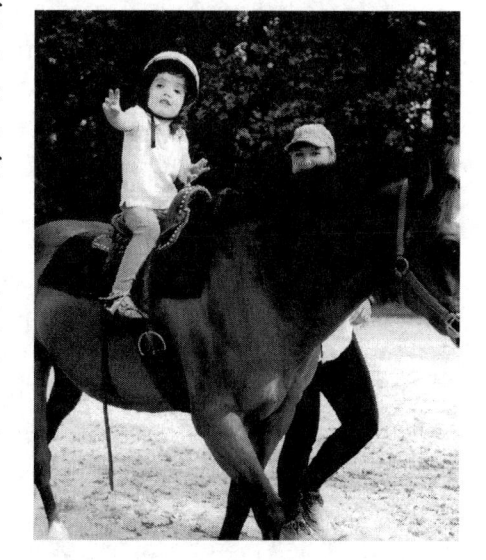

***

While we are not advocating buying a pony for all disabled children, our message is to "think outside the box" for the physically challenged child. When mobility from young age is limited, it is *paramount* that some form of physical activity be pursued for the child. Empowerment for the child and parents can help to guide the child to a more active future lifestyle.

Many federal and state resources are available to better understand what the child with disabilities is entitled to receive. The Social Security Office and your state's office of Medicaid are good places to start for more information. These services can sometimes provide therapists who can help improve physical assistance and mobility for the child or adult with disabilities. These resources can likewise also help provide assistance with the person's nutritional needs.

What are the Nutritional Limitations?
- Has the child been evaluated by a speech therapist?
- What are the dietary restrictions?
- Does the individual have proper teeth and dentition?
- Does he or she require a soft or liquid diet?
- Is TPN (Total Parenteral Nutrition) needed (more likely for an in-patient individual)?
- Does the individual receive food through a feeding tube? PEG tube or J-Tube?

Referral to a nutritionist is a high priority in the case of an individual with disabilities, especially if he or she has impaired feeding ability and/or changes in caloric requirements. Speech therapists are great resources for evaluating feeding needs, which is something not everyone thinks about (not even all medical people seem to realize this).

Does the individual in question require a swallow study to monitor safe swallowing of water versus thickened liquids?

Remember that, for a child with disabilities, challenges often continue throughout life. But, sometimes they change, which requires a continued focus on maintaining adequate nutrition and eating safety. Voicing to the caregiver that you understand the stress of safely providing the best nutrition possible for a child or adult with disabilities can help assure the caregiver.

Balanced nutrition is essential for people with disabilities, since there are so many other challenges they must face. Providing a stress-free environment for eating is also crucial for children with disabilities, because they sometimes feel the stress that can surround their eating, whether they eat "too much" or "too little." Remember that, for a person with disabilities, food should be provided in a relaxed environment and can provide an opportunity for learning, comfort, and social bonding. (And you may want to consider making mealtimes with anyone, disabled or not, as relaxed as possible, for the very same reasons.)

***

DEBBIE'S STORY *(continued)*: My daughter has had a complicated course with nutritional needs. Beginning with failure to thrive from difficulty nursing and feeding from a young age, she has had many eating issues relating to facial paralysis and dental abnormalities. She has had ongoing speech therapy and oral motor therapy.

Despite craniofacial challenges, she has compensated remarkably well and loves to eat a wide variety of foods. (She has a very mature palate for spicy and ethnic foods.) Though she was on a calcium-restricted diet for years due to *excess* calcium in her bones, she still enjoyed pizza (stripped of cheese) and vegetarian cheeses.

She recently required a swallow study that demonstrated narrowing and stricture of the esophagus, which delayed swallowing. The question became: how do I continue to give her the nutrition she needs in the safest possible way? One recommendation was to encourage sips of drink between bites of food. (Yes, something as simple as this can help.) And while she enjoys steak, giving her meat in the form of a burger or braised meat makes it safer for her to ingest.

At the pediatrician's office a week ago, my daughter told the nurse that I was being a "Jewish Mother" since I was concerned that she had lost twelve pounds. Jokingly, I told her that I would definitely make her matzo ball soup, a classic Jewish food. And I did – which she ate very well. She enjoyed carrots, potatoes, zucchini, celery, parsnip, chicken and onions (and a few secret ingredients!). She helped me wash the vegetables, and we had a cultural discussion of food and family along the way.

***

Disability and the Workforce

The majority of this chapter has focused on children with disabilities. Yet these children will eventually become adults with disabilities. Whether or not they become mainstreamed, working members of society, they will continue to be impaired in one way or another. Whether or not they spend their day working, or at a Day Center of some sort, they will continue with the same challenges (and more) of the typical, sedentary workforce in the United States.

Desk jobs and busy schedules limit the ability of people to get outdoors, become active, or make certain nutrition choices. This is why *corporate wellness* has become such a growing field. People who work in this field provide health programs or incentives to eat well and remain active; these programs may ultimately improve wellness of the workforce, while also saving costs on healthcare.

Recognizing how challenging it can be to maintain corporate wellness among non-disabled individuals, we need to understand the difficulties with regards to adults with disabilities. With already limited mobility, many adults with disabilities cannot work and have the potential for further health complications.

According to Healthy People 2020:
- 14.5 percent of people with disabilities were unemployed in 2009.
- 19.2 percent of people with disabilities were employed in 2009.
  (The goal of Healthy People 2020 is to better the percentage by 10%.)

Disability statistics from 2010 indicate that 31% of adults aged 18 to 64 with work limitations were living below the poverty line (Nazarov & Lee, 2012). This is based on the current population survey, in which a disability was defined as a "health problem or disability which prevents them from working or which limits the kind or amount of work they can do" (Nazarov & Lee, 2012). Despite the exact type of disability, we must appreciate that not only are so many Americans disabled in some way (which can limit their physical ability to work), but they also are living with fewer economic resources (thus increasing their likelihood of "falling through the cracks" in the system). Note that these surveys are, at best, a sampling of reported people with disabilities. Nurses must recognize that many people, for various reasons, are either undiagnosed, unreported, or lack access to care. How can nurses encourage health promotion and preventative care among this population?

Many state and federal programs exist for adults with disabilities. Unfortunately, in today's financial climate, much of the funding has been reduced for people with disabilities. Not only do adults with congenital disabilities struggle with health and obesity, but now we have a surging population of people who are becoming disabled due to obesity, diabetes, or other related conditions. This means that society will now have to deal seriously with the compounded issues of the disabled workforce.

Summary

Every child with disabilities is unique, and has unique nutritional needs. But all of this should fall within the framework of balanced nutrition (which we encourage as a goal for everyone). As there are more people with disabilities than ever before, there is likely to be an increase in the number of people with disabilities who are overweight or obese as well.

Because of this, there will be more and more people with underlying disabilities being diagnosed with diabetes and other nutrition-related conditions. Nutritional education for people with disabilities is now more important than ever, because disability and obesity will compound the risks and complications of each condition.

Caring for a child or adult with disabilities is challenging enough as it is. Encouraging the need for continued, sustained and balanced nutrition – and activity – for the person with disabilities is paramount to overall health.

As a nurse, parents will often look to you for guidance. What can you do to encourage children with disabilities to access and share in wellness and health activities?

1. **Encourage parents not to be shy.** Tell them to take their disabled child to a public or private wellness place. Is there a local YMCA or community center? Most non-profit programs, such as United Way (or programs funded by United Way) must follow the Individuals with Disabilities Act rules of providing access to people with disabilities (ramps, elevators, lifts, widened doors, etc.). One of the biggest barriers is the confidence of the parent or caregiver to feel that it's okay to mainstream the child, even if he/she cannot function the same as non-impaired children.
2. **Provide a referral** or sounding board for the parent or guardian. National Dissemination Center for Children with Disabilities lists organizations by state, and can help direct you to local programs: http://nichcy.org/.
3. Invite a caregiver or friend to join at an IEP (Individual Education Plan) meeting to help **advocate for the child**. Remember, the child is entitled to the *"least restrictive environment,"* which includes school P.E. classes.
4. Explain how limited mobility can lead to weight gain and other related issues.
5. **Refer the family to nutrition services** to monitor caloric needs. Remind them that "calories in, calories out" is the balance between food and beverages consumed, and the activities that help burn the

---

NOTE: If there are medical reasons for a restricted diet, the parents should understand the new diet in the context of a typical balanced diet. If the child receives a mechanical soft (blended) diet, the same needs can be fulfilled by balancing fruits, vegetables, grains, and protein. Extra care should be made to monitor the diet, so the foods being used are not all processed and high in sodium.

---

6. Encourage use of **physical therapy**, as most therapists have very good knowledge of exercises appropriate for different levels of ability.

7. Help **involve the child** with disabilities to participate in **food preparation and/or purchase** to provide a good learning environment.
8. Help **expose the person with disabilities to new foods and activities**. Encourage new exploration of food through touching, feeling, and tasting.

These are just a few pointers to help the parents of children with disabilities navigate what is a lifelong, and often confusing, path. Care, patience, and compassion will go a long way, even if the nurse is not fully knowledgeable regarding the exact disability. Continued care of a child with disabilities to adulthood is challenging, but monitoring that they continue to progress emotionally, physically, and medically is necessary.

References

Brault, M. (2005). Americans with Disabilities:, Current Population Reports, pp 70-107, U.S. Census Bureau, Washington, DC. 2008. Retrieved 04/12/12 from http://www.census.gov/prod/2008pubs/p70-117.pdf

Doody, C.M. and Doody, O. (2012). Health promotion for people with intellectual disability and obesity. *British Journal of Nursing*, Apr 26-May 9, pp 460, 462-5.

Erickson, W., Lee, C., von Schrader, S. (2012). Disability Statistics from the 2010 American Community Survey (ACS). Ithaca, NY: Cornell University Rehabilitation Research and Training Center on Disability Demographics and Statistics (StatsRRTC). Retrieved 07/04/12 from www.disabilitystatistics.org

Nazarov, Z., Lee, C. G. (2012). *Disability Statistics from the Current Population Survey (CPS)*. Ithaca, NY: Cornell University Rehabilitation Research and Training Center on Disability Demographics and Statistics (StatsRRTC). Retrieved 07/04/12 from www.disabilitystatistics.org

Nazarov, Z., Lee, C. G. (2012). *Disability Statistics from the Current Population Survey (CPS)*. Ithaca, NY: Cornell University Rehabilitation Research and Training Center on Disability Demographics and Statistics (StatsRRTC). Retrieved 07/04/12 from www.disabilitystatistics.org

Reinehr, T., Dobe, M., Winkel, K., Schaefer, A. and Hoffmann, D. (2010). Obesity in Disabled Children and Adolescents An Overlooked Group of Patients, *Deutsches Arzteblatt International*. doi: 10.3238/arztebl.2010.0268. Retrieved 04/26/12 from http://www.ncbi.nlm.nih.gov/pmc/articles/PMC2864441/

United States Census Bureau (2005). Americans with Disabilities 2005. Retrieved 04/13/12 from http://www.census.gov/hhes/www/disability/sipp/disable05.html

United States Department of Health and Human Services (HHS), (2012), *Disability and Health*. Retrieved 04/13/12 from http://healthypeople.gov/2020/topicsobjectives2020/objectiveslist.aspx?topicId=9

PART III: ASSESSMENT

In Parts I and II, we identified social and cultural health indicators, learned how to take a health history, and explored physical exam findings related to obesity. In Part III, we combine what we know thus far and assess the "big picture." Nurses must understand how obesity and related conditions can affect each patient uniquely. How does weight status or obesity affect *this patient*, given the individual health indicators and clinical history? WHO is our patient and WHAT are their needs? By determining health indicators related to obesity and how to clinically assess the individual patient, we have only *begun* the process that leads to successful health interventions. Without an ASSESSMENT phase of the obesity prevention strategy, we as nurses would fail to set goals for and implement an actual plan for our patient. The assessment portion requires nurses to use **critical thinking skills** and **good judgment** to assess the comprehensive and multidisciplinary components of our patient's heathcare needs. This phase of full understanding is needed to develop the plan in Part IV.

This portion of the guide includes chapters that explain the following:
- **Chapter 7: Know Your Patient: Health Assessment**
- **Chapter 8: Adolescence, Health & Obesity**
- **Chapter 9: Adult Health & Obesity**
- **Chapter 10: Maternal Health & Obesity**
- **Chapter 11: Obesity & Older Adults**

This section will expand on the first two parts of the Guide to better understand the significant health risks of obesity within each stage of development.

Part III Objectives:

1. Outline how obesity affects health during different stages of development
2. Classify gender differences and health needs at different ages
3. Recognize the complexity of obesity related to adult health

Chapter 7
Know Your Patient: Health Assessment

In this chapter, we discuss typical growth and milestones of children. Although there is some normal variability in the development of children, we can use healthy or normal parameters to anticipate, prevent, and manage the risk of childhood obesity in its early stages. Like rings of tree bark, our bodies undergo set patterns by which our growth, age, and developmental stages can be monitored. Throughout our lives, our bodies develop along a typical path, and the typical trends provide us with milestones by which to monitor age-appropriate developmental growth in children. The first five years of life mark the most rapid and substantial changes in the development of the human body.

Despite the use of milestones and parameters, nurses must also recognize the normal variability in growth and development. As with any other portion of the nursing assessment process, understanding the "normal" findings can help one understand what is not a normal path of growth and development, even for a unique individual. Thus, growth charts should be used only as a guide, because each individual child grows at a slightly different rate (along his or her own growth curve) than every other child.

> Chapter 7 Objectives:
> 1. Explain the typical growth milestones for children
> 2. Illustrate how growth and development affect the child's nutritional and fitness needs
> 3. Differentiate between male and female growth and development
> 4. Describe how growth and development affect future health

What are the typical growth milestones for children?

Understanding how the social and physical determinants affect vulnerable individuals from *birth* through old age is important when we look at health promotion and habits even from a young age. Before infants are born, they are monitored for growth and compared to standards of size and weight. Within minutes of the infant's birth, his or her weight and length are taken, and an APGAR score is given to determine the initial health of the baby. Then, basic measurements are recorded. At this point, various questions emerge, such as: is the child longer or shorter than average? Is the infant heavier or lighter than average? Does the child's head circumference match the expected size compared to the weight and length of the child? (We know, for example, that infants of mothers with diabetes are often born with high birth weights, though this does not doom them to a later diagnosis of diabetes.)

The next question is, *"what do all these measurements mean for the child?"* While the length and weight of a baby are not necessarily predicative of later measurements, the growth pattern of the infant throughout childhood will be used to monitor his or her growth along the expected "growth curve."

A multitude of researchers have developed many different parameters by which to monitor how children grow and develop along an expected trajectory. As with any component of a physical exam, the *baseline* of the individual patient is crucial. Clinicians must compare the child not only to his or her *unique* baseline, but then also consider the standardized, accepted "normal" measurements and developmental milestones. Whether the clinician uses the Denver Developmental Exam or a comparable standard of measurement, the clinician monitors whether progress has been made and whether or not the child has continued his or her due growth. (For example, a clinician might ask himself, "is there a delay in this child's growth?" "Is the child reaching milestones early?" Or, "is the child's growth right with the growth chart in all parameters," – with this last being what all parents hope for.) Based on these considerations, the nurse and staff can help the family understand the child's needs.

We know that babies are dependent from birth. Their needs for nutrition are high and their metabolism is high, but they do not really *do* much of anything. Infants drink (milk or formula), they burp, they cry, they wiggle, and they eliminate their waste. Though all of this sounds simple, infants quickly progress in a typical way. Every one or two months during their first year, children become more accomplished. Most find their mouths within a few weeks, start paying attention to the outside world, and gradually become more mobile by crawling, then walking. And all of this occurs within the first year.

During this time, the caregiver, parents (mother and father), guardian, or nurse has established a pattern of care for the expected needs for the infant. For example, "Is the child active?" "Is he or she often left alone?" "Is the child always helped, or is he or she expected to manage, somehow, alone?" "Is the child encouraged to crawl, or later, walk?" And the last question, which has been a hotbed of contention for years: "Is the child breastfed, bottle-fed, or a combination of both?"

> **NOTE:** Although typically considered immunologically and even intellectually beneficial for infants, many sources debate how significant and long-term the effects breast feeding are on a child as compared to their bottle-fed counterparts. We make no judgment either way. Our goal is to promote the best choices and best health, given the opportunities available. We hope that each parent will become empowered through health literacy to decide what is best, and to understand which resources are within their reach for health promotion and support.

It is essential to understand that, by the age of eighteen months, children have the ability and capacity to be active and to start feeding themselves. Toddlers at eighteen months should be able to drink from a cup, feed themselves with a spoon, pretend play by feeding dolls, walk (including up steps), and maybe even run (CDC). As you see, children who are eighteen months old *already*, if given the right environment, have the necessary means to stay active and eat well.

Along with charting the growth, feeding, and sleeping patterns of the child, a clinician monitors how well that child interacts within his environment (at least as far as the office environment, where the child is likely to be assessed). The clinician may ask, *"Does the child make eye contact with people around him?" "Does she reach out for toys?" "Does he feed?"*

Which raises the following questions: will the child who can feed himself have the proper nutrition at his fingertips? And will the child be given the opportunities to be active and explore her environment? If not, we (as nurses) need to focus our immediate attention on the caregiver in order to start giving proper health education as soon as possible.

Helping the caregiver to understand what the milestones are, and why they are important, will enable and encourage the caregiver to help *advocate* for the child during times when the child cannot yet advocate for himself. And you, the nurse, can emphasize that the early physical and social environments to which a toddler is exposed (whether at home, school, or in the community) can set the stage for the child's future habits.

A Healthy People 2020 paper on social determinants clearly explains that achieving health is far more complex than just preventing and treating illness (HHS & USDA, 2010). Nurses need to understand how the child's physical and social environments can affect progression through appropriate developmental milestones. (As with anything, the standard "growth curve" will only get you so far.) For instance, by age five, for a child to be considered fully and physically developed, he or she should be able to hop, skip and do a somersault. Questions to ask are: Is the child given opportunities to grow and change? Is he or she given opportunities to run around and play? All of these questions need to be considered in order to fully understand why some milestones may be "hit" – and why some may not be.

1. **How does growth and development affect the child's nutritional and fitness needs?**

The fastest physical growth occurs during the first five years of life. During this time of rapid skull growth, the fontanelles close, long bones lengthen, and the soft bones harden. Muscles continue to develop as children become more mobile and use their bodies more. By age five, a child has all twenty deciduous or "milk" teeth, thus enabling more chewing and grinding, and a better ability to eat.

With rapid growth, there is a high metabolic demand, but also specific nutritional needs. The caloric requirements of a child are high, but they are not the same as a fully-grown adult. And, while certain requirements are needed, such as full fat (whole) milk until age two, this does not mean that a child should ingest a high calorie and high fat diet.

Nurses, parents, and children should all recognize that **children are not small adults**. If we ignore the different needs of children compared to adults, we jeopardize their movement through appropriate milestones and developmental growth. Children have specific caloric and nutritional requirements, just as they require medication doses tapered for their weight.

Whether or not you are a pediatric nurse, you likely remember your pediatric rotation when you practiced calculating pediatric medication dosages. As annoying as the math calculations seemed at the time, it was necessary to not accidentally *overdose* a child. Similarly, since "calories in, calories out" is the mantra to balance energy intake (calories) and energy output (activity/fitness), we must taper the food intake for children, so they don't *overdose*.

Recognizing that children have food interests different than those of adults is important, but we must also understand the amount and characteristics of foods that interest children. Feeding a child an adult-sized portion, whether at home or in a restaurant, is not appropriate for his or her caloric needs. Unfortunately, many of the kid-sized meals, though smaller in portion, contain just as many calories as a good choice off the adult menu. This is why you may be better off to help a child select a healthier choice off the adult menu, then ask for a child-sized portion, than allow that child to order from the attractively-packaged kid's menu.

Parental food choice will often influence a child's food choice, and there's nothing wrong with that as far as it goes. The problem comes in when parents choose foods for their child without understanding how diverse a palate a child can have.

A study from the Cornell Foods and Brand Lab demonstrated that children, compared to their adult counterparts, actually prefer a wider variety of foods. Despite popular belief, children actually *choose* more colorful foods and more variety (seven different foods and six colors of food on one plate) than their adult counterparts (three foods and three colors on one plate) (Zampollo et al., 2012). This bodes well for the USDA recommendations on food variety and colors, but we must be sure that the colors are not from artificially colored sugared cereals when they could be from fresh fruit instead.

To promote adequate growth and development, children require a balanced diet to help provide the many vitamins and minerals necessary for growth. The following chart shows some basic vitamins children should consume on a regular basis.

Table 7-1. VITAMINS FOR GROWTH

VITAMIN	NEEDED FOR	SAMPLE FOODS
Vitamin A	For healthy bones, skin, hair, nails, vision	Carrots, cantaloupe, grapefruit, papaya, squash, sweet potatoes, tomatoes, watermelon, pecans
B Vitamins Including B9 (folate) and B12	Formation of red blood cells, metabolism of food, normal brain function	Fish, meat, cheese, eggs, wheat, fruits and vegetables
Vitamin C	Antioxidant and immune function	Citrus, berries, leafy greens, fish
Vitamin D	Health of teeth and bones, calcium, magnesium and phosphorus absorption	sunshine, yogurt, cheese, fish, beef
Vitamin E	Antioxidant, skin and brain health	Berries, squash, nuts, fish, meat
Vitamin K	Blood clotting and bone health	Many berries, leafy vegetables, meats, cheese

© 2012 HERO Inc.

Following the guidelines at USDA Choosemyplate.gov will help one plan proper meals for children.

Nurses and parents alike must remember the influence they have over children and their choices. When they see you eating a healthy choice, they will be more likely to try it as well. Unfortunately, some parents are so busy with daily life that convenience often outweighs the parent's ability to make a wise choice for not only themselves, but for their children as well. Helping parents to understand the basic importance of nutrition can encourage improved habits; highlight the main categories of food, and how parents can incorporate them into their busy daily schedule, to obtain the best results.

7: *Know Your Patient: Health Assessment*

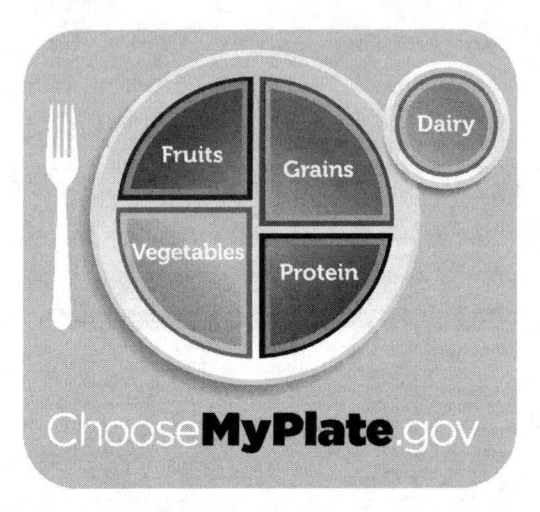

Figure 7-1. USDA Food Choice Illustration (2012)
Reprinted with permission by USDA.

To help summarize the USDA recommendations for healthy eating, the HERO program created the summary table below.

Table 7-2. FOOD GROUPS

MAIN FOOD GROUPS	WHY	HOW MUCH (DEPENDENT ON AGE AND GENDER, WITH BOYS NEEDING MORE BY AGE 18)	HOW
FRUITS	Vitamins, minerals, antioxidants, water, fiber	1-2 cups a day	Fresh is best. Frozen, canned, or dried unsweetened
VEGETABLES	Vitamins, minerals, fiber, water, antioxidants	1-3 cups a day	Fresh is best. Frozen, canned, or baked. Fried is least healthy
GRAINS	Vitamins, minerals, protein, fiber, iron. Whole grains help to reduce cholesterol and reduce constipation.	3-8 ounces a day (1 slice of bread~ 1 ounce)	Choose whole grains when possible for more fiber. The darker and less processed the bread or pasta, the better.

(Continued)

FOOD GROUPS *(continued)*			
MAIN FOOD GROUPS	**WHY**	**HOW MUCH (DEPENDENT ON AGE AND GENDER, WITH BOYS NEEDING MORE BY AGE 18)**	**HOW**
PROTEINS	Protein for muscle, red blood cells, iron. Helps you feel full longer. Energy with fewer empty calories	2-6.5 ounces (1 can tuna= 5 ounces)	Choose lean and less processed meats and fish. Canned fish is a good alternative. Beans and nuts.
DAIRY	Protein, calcium, vitamin D, for bone development and strength. Until age 2: drink whole milk	2-3 cups daily	Low fat or non-fat milk, cheese, and yogurt.

© 2012 HERO Inc.

While we have heard time and time again that we need 8 glasses of water a day, this is rarely included in tables. (Notice that the USDA does not include a glass of water as part of a healthy plate.) To emphasize that water is the most necessary and best beverage, HERO includes water as a "group" unto itself.

Table 7-3. WATER

WATER	Hydrate skin; 70% of body is water	8 glasses/day	Water, and unsweetened drinks

© 2012 HERO Inc.

Let us not forget *four* categories of concern:

Table 7-4. FOODS TO EAT IN MODERATION

FATS/OILS	High in calories, contribute to high cholesterol and weight gain	Monounsaturated fats and omega3s are good fats in nuts, avocados, olive oil. Other fats should be limited.	Saturated fats: French fries, hamburgers, cookies, cakes, salad dressing
SUGARS	High in calories, contribute to weight gain and tooth decay	Limit empty calories. Replace with natural sugars like honey, natural sugars from fruit	Also in French fries and breads. "empty calories" provide no nutrients
ALCOHOL	High in calories, contributes to liver disease, impaired judgment and safety	Small amounts of alcohol (4 oz. of wine, one to two 12-oz. beers) may aid in digestion. Please drink responsibly.	Under age 21, drinking is illegal in the United States. Children and young adults under this age should avoid alcohol.
SALT	Contributes to heart disease and high blood pressure, dehydrates	<2,300 mg/day or 1 teaspoon/day. Sea salt is lower in sodium than table salt. Avoid adding additional salt to foods. Try pepper, salsa, lemon, herbs instead	Prepared foods, some low-fat foods add salt to improve taste. The more processed the food, the higher it is in sodium

© 2012 HERO Inc.

Due to the decline in eating fresh foods, fruits, and vegetables, many children do not eat the foods needed for healthy bodies. While it is always best to obtain needed vitamins from the original food source, supplemental vitamins are a good secondary option. Just remember that oral vitamins are not absorbed as well as foods, do not contain other nutrients like fiber that are necessary for proper digestion, and do not help encourage healthy eating patterns.

We point this out because if a child eats mostly fast food, but takes a daily vitamin, he might believe that his pattern of eating is sufficient because of the vitamin supplementation. This would be shortsighted, as he will still be likely ingesting too many empty calories, which lack fundamental nutrients.

2. How and why do we continue to monitor growth and development?

Pediatricians and nurses continue to monitor a child's growth to determine if the child continues to grow along the expected growth trajectory. Charts like the CDC growth charts are routinely used to monitor for *continuous* and *normal* growth. The questions these charts tend to answer are these: where does the child fall among his or her peers? Is he/she among the shorter and heavier, or taller and thinner group? If there is a change in his established growth pattern, what is the possible cause? Have eating habits changed, is there underlying illness, or is there possibly a developmental reason for a change?

Since childhood and adolescence are the times of most rapid growth, we assume that beyond those critical years, weight and certainly height remain somewhat constant. Thus, clinicians may abandon the use of growth measurements in favor of other clinical assessment tools. But, today more than ever, continuing to monitor BMI, height, weight, even waist size is necessary to face the challenges of increased childhood obesity that continues into adulthood.

We will continue to see a shift in *where* and *how* this health (growth and development) monitoring occurs. Given recent trends in health policies, it is plausible that monitoring of growth will shift more to schools and community settings. Already, many schools have certain requirements regarding monitoring height, weight, and BMI via the school nurse. In today's healthcare climate, where health insurance costs are high, and access is readily available for all, there must be a greater focus on health promotion and *consistent* monitoring of growth. Though this guide explains HOW to measure BMI and WHY we need to, there remain significant gaps in the reality of "what happens next."

3. What are the differences between male and female growth and development?

We know that clearly men and women are very different, not only physically but also psychosocially, and their different patterns of growth and development contribute to these distinct differences. Notoriously, even from conception, people pride themselves on being able to decide whether a pregnant mother is carrying a boy or a girl. How low, wide, high, or round the pregnant belly may be, people recognize that already there are male and female differences. Even the heart rate of a male versus female fetus can differ (the male heart might beat slightly slower).

Clearly, the greatest differences between boys and girls *before* the onset of puberty are the genital differences. Otherwise, boys and girls *before* puberty tend to grow and develop at relatively constant and similar rates. Bone growth, including the long bones, closure of infant skull fontanelles, and tooth development are comparable for boys and girls. And even physical and psychosocial developmental milestones for boys and girls of this age are mostly the same.

One study by Harbaugh et al. (2011) researched the number of overweight and obese low income Mississippi preschoolers in 2005 and 2010 (with identical methods). Findings showed that rates of obesity were 20.6% and 20.8% obese, respectively in 2005 and 2010, which was not statistically significant and appeared to mimic a stabilizing trend among low income preschoolers. There were no differences among race or gender at this age. This has implications for group teaching and the need to educate all children regardless of race and socioeconomic status.

Diagnostic health assessment tools, such as the Denver Developmental Screening Test, do not discern between male and female gender when assessing children between the ages of 0 and 6 years old (Cadman et al., 1988). And such a test is deemed an appropriate means to monitor future health risk of both boys and girls alike. This highlights the need for early intervention for boys and girls at a time when they are first developing. Using appropriate diagnostic screening tools, and before further intrinsic and extrinsic factors make growth and development even more complicated, educators and nurses can collaborate to help improve future health and reduce obesity.

To understand how early intervention and awareness of obesity at a young age can be effective, we must ponder a few questions:

- What are the practical implications of gender differences at a young age?
- Can girls and boys at a young age begin to learn health education effectively?
- Can girls and boys learn health education together in a class setting?

> While working with 6 year-old students, our HERO program demonstrated successfully that educating girls and boys together effectively empowered all children. There were no gender differences in terms of interest, participation, ability, or retention of information. We also found subjectively that, at a young age of 6, there were no racial differences in terms of participation or even rates of obesity among higher and lower socioeconomic status. Though we have not to date formally studied this, we certainly find a need to pursue formal research to promote the need for early intervention by age 6, across both genders, and all socioeconomic groups and races.

No doubt obesity rates are dramatically high even among young boys and girls, and nurses must understand how to incorporate knowledge of developmental stage and gender differences at any stage of growth. Of course, as children age, the methods of providing health education will evolve, as gender differences such as physical ability, strength, caloric needs, interests increase.

By age 10, the developmental differences begin to diverge, as girls develop faster, marked by earlier changes in genitalia, hormones, and then menstruation (which of course boys will never have). Menarche often begins by age 12 or 13 (now earlier than a century ago when onset began around 15 or 16), 3 years earlier than the start of male pubescent changes. Boys also demonstrate significant increase in growth, with inches add to their height and increased muscle mass, and therefore have higher caloric needs than girls at a similar age. Hormonal changes contribute to genital growth and increased hair growth. Becoming familiar with the stages of sexual maturity is significant because the rise in obesity is changing how quickly children develop, and nurses might observe signs of sexual maturity on physical exam at younger ages than decades ago.

The Tanner Stages of Sexual Maturity has been the gold standard by which to measure growth according to pubic hair and genitalia. For example, the chart below summarizes maturity stages of female breast and male genitalia.

Table 7-5. SEXUAL MATURITY

Female Breast	Sexual Maturity	Hair Growth
Raised nipple, No breast bud	I	No hair
Breast bud	II	Sparse hair
Raised mound	III	More hair, more coarse
Enlargement of nipple, and areola as mound	IV	Adult pubic hair, not to thighs
Mature breast with areola contouring the breast	V	Adult hair spread to medial thighs

Male Genitalia	Sexual Maturity	Hair Growth
Early childhood size, No growth	I	No hair
Enlargement of scrotum and testes, reddening of scrotal skin	II	Sparse hair
Growth in length, width of penis shaft	III	More hair, more coarse
Growth of scrotum, penis and testes, darkening of skin	IV	Adult hair, not to thighs
Adult genitalia	V	Adult hair spread to medial thighs

© 2012 HERO Inc.

Adapted from Tanner JM. Growth at adolescence. Oxford: Blackwell Scientific Publications, 1962.

Although these dramatic body and developmental changes occur at puberty, in the teenage years, research in the context of childhood obesity now demonstrates how the timing of puberty can be influenced by the growth and development of boys and girls even during the early years (when gender differences were not otherwise as marked). Whereas childhood obesity during the first few years for boys was found to cause *delayed* puberty (in 14% of boys with higher BMI), childhood obesity among U.S. girls (measured by elevated BMI by age 36 months and until first grade) was found to cause *earlier* onset of puberty (Lee et. al. 2010, Lee et. al. 2007, respectively). By middle school years, children know they will be separated by gender to discuss sex education. The girls will discuss pregnancy, menstruation, and use of sanitary products. And the boys will discuss use of a condom, ejaculation, and use of deodorant. But nutritional and health needs of the adolescent are not adequately discussed.

Health education for adolescents must highlight the male/female differences, not only related to genital and sexual changes, but also related the different caloric and exercise needs of males and females, as these differences will continue.

The following calorie chart shows the daily caloric needs by age but also by gender. Note how dramatic the differences are between female and male teenage needs. The needs of a girl are sometimes only 75% of the boys' needs. This is very significant. Despite the different caloric needs, there are no separate "boy meals" and "girl meals." We easily forget that, boys and girls (and men and women) are so very different; there is a continued attempt to equalize our needs. As boys and girls grow and develop, their metabolic, physical, and anatomical characteristics change considerably. Just as "one size does *not* fit all," we need to consider any specific needs for boys versus girls. A twelve-year-old boy during puberty has higher caloric requirements, and more rapid growth, than a fourteen-year-old boy who has not yet begun pubertal changes. Assessing and monitoring growth and nutritional requirements for children should be done on an individual basis according to their history of growth and development.

Below is a caloric intake chart that explains the needs of children according to age and gender (Male and female caloric requirements vary considerably beyond age nine; keep this in mind.):

Table 7-6. CALORIC NEEDS BY AGE

AGE	CALORIC NEED
0 to 6 months	55kcal/lb
6 months to 1 year	45 kcal/lb
Toddler 1-3	850-1300 kcal/day
4 to 8	1400-2000
9 to 13	BOYS: 1800-2600/day
	GIRLS: 1600-2000/day
Teenager	20 kcal/lb
	BOYS: 2800-3200/day
	GIRLS: 2400/day

© 2012 HERO Inc.

4. How does growth and development affect future health?

The need to monitor growth and development related to *typical* development and *typical* gender growth differences and caloric requirements were discussed in the previous sections. In addition to the possibility of early obesity leading to early or late onset of adolescence (depending on gender and other factors), how else does growth (and obesity) affect future health?

Continued monitoring of growth and development sets the stage for continued health promotion to ensure that children do follow the appropriate continuum of development, which ultimately can lead to better long-term health. Again, we cannot ignore the complex issues of nature versus nurture, but to give children their best opportunities for a life free of illness, we must monitor and understand how growth and the possibility of obesity affects children, adolescence, and the entire lifespan.

With the rise in childhood obesity, more and more medical conditions are now being linked to obesity. A recent Swedish study followed 2075 children over eight years and found that children with a high BMI at age seven were more likely to have asthma. But if children with a high BMI before age seven reduced their BMI to normal by age seven, they had no greater risk of developing asthma (Magnusson, 2011). This shows the need to monitor BMI and the weight of a young child during the first few years of life. (Until recently, the majority of BMI studies have been conducted on older children.) Whether obesity can increase the chances of earlier diagnosis or long-term chances of asthma, heart disease, joint disease, or more, EARLY INTERVENTION, EDUCATION, and PREVENTION of obesity must be a targeted focus of growth and development education.

The CDC continues to improve health policies to pave the way for continued growth monitoring. In 2005, the CDC developed guidelines for use of BMI screenings in schools. There still remains controversy about the efficacy of, and best ways to implement, such programs. There are fears that students' privacy will be compromised and students will become stigmatized, and there is a distinct lack of support services for those with high BMI and who are at risk of obesity.

In theory, a school environment with proper support services and staff training would be a natural means of monitoring children's growth throughout their primary years. However, without appropriate follow-up services, a system of screening can only be so effective. Because so few states and cities have yet to implement school-based BMI and health screening programs, it remains for the pediatrician to properly monitor the growth and development of the child. Nurses can help raise awareness of the need for "well visits" with pediatricians so they can monitor growth and development.

Over time, well visits to pediatricians have been the mainstay for monitoring the growth and development of children. The height, weight, and growth of children are measured in many different ways and then are recorded on the children's health charts. Pediatricians clearly are the health promotion providers needed for consistent care. However, what measures are taken to follow through if a patient is at risk for obesity? The issue of childhood obesity is a somewhat gray area, neither part of a sick visit or well visit. Children at risk of obesity require more health promotion and counseling than a typical child visiting the doctor annually. Yet, without an explicit diagnosis or illness, those children might not receive the needed nutrition counseling. And the parents likely are not fully aware of the health implications of their children's obesity or risk of obesity.

Rising childhood obesity rates show there is a need for expanded health promotion by nurses. Right now, there is little intervention given at the earliest possible stages in order to reduce – or possibly prevent – obesity in children. Nurses must help prioritize early intervention and help raise awareness of obesity and increased risk of hypertension, diabetes, asthma, and more – even among youth.

Among the children affected by obesity, there is a significant health disparity. Socioeconomic status, race, ethnicity, and gender all demonstrate differences in rates of obesity. Clearly, this Guide highlights the fact that childhood obesity has increased dramatically over the past three decades. But we must also understand the specific trends in order to understand what can be done about it. Statistics demonstrate that ALL sectors of the population have their share of obesity rates, and these rates are increasing across all races, age groups, and even socioeconomic groups.

There will soon be less of a disparity among races, as White American children are seeing higher rates of obesity, though rates among Black and Hispanic Americans are still higher and climbing. From 1976 to 2007, the total percentage of children ages 6 to 17 who are obese has risen from 5.2% to 19.2% (National Center for Health Statistics, 2010). The obesity rates among White American children tripled from 4.9% to 17.4% since 1976, and obesity among Black Americans nearly tripled from 8.2% to 22.4%. Hispanic Americans, with no available statistics in 1976, in 2007 had the highest rates of child obesity, at 24.2%. And Hispanics are less likely to receive counseling on healthy eating and exercise. Still now, we see that older adults are more likely to a) be told they are overweight and b) be given counseling on what to do about it. The need for identifying, addressing, and educating youth from an early age is critical.

While the prevalence of obesity has clearly increased over the past three decades, the disparity among socioeconomic status has declined. A study by Zhang and Wang (2004) used data from National Health and Nutrition Examination Surveys (NHANES) to analyze over 28,000 people (ages 20 to 60) between 1971 and 2000. While the relative difference in disparity among three socioeconomic groups (low, medium, and high) was 50% in 1971, it decreased to a relative disparity of 14% by 2000. Study findings conclude that socio-environmental influences appear greater than individual characteristics of the person. This means that, although lower socioeconomic status often increases the risk of disease processes for a variety of reasons, no cohort is immune to obesity, even among higher socioeconomic groups. This emphasizes the need to provide education and intervention across ALL socioeconomic groups. This is why our HERO program, though focusing initially on lower socioeconomic groups, provides outreach to communities at large. HERO recognizes that obesity does not occur in a vacuum, nor can anyone become immune to it. Intervention must be offered to all, though greater intervention is required for those with more contributing factors.

The following charts by the CDC show the percentage of children who were told by a doctor that they are overweight or obese children. Other charts show the percentage of children who received advice by the doctor regarding nutrition and physical activity.

7: Know Your Patient: Health Assessment

Table 7-7. Percentage of children and adolescents ages 6-17 who are obese by race/Hispanic origin. (2007-2008)

African American	White, Non-Hispanic	African American: White, Non-Hispanic Ratio
22.4	17.4	1.3

Source: Federal Interagency Forum on Child and Family Statistics. America's Children: Key National Indicators of well-Being. 2010. Reprinted with permission from CDC.gov. (National Center for Health Statistics, 2010)

Table 7-8. Percentage of obese children and teens ages 2-19 who were told by a doctor that they were overweight, 2003-2006

Non-Hispanic Black	Non-Hispanic White	Non-Hispanic Black/ Non-Hispanic White Ratio
44.4	36.9	1.2

Source: 2009 National Healthcare Disparities Report. Reprinted with permission from CDC.gov. (HHS and AHRQ, 2009)

Table 7-9. Percent of children ages 2-17 for whom a doctor or other health provider ever gave advice about amount/kind of physical activity, United States, 2006

Non-Hispanic Black	Non-Hispanic White	Non-Hispanic Black/ Non-Hispanic White Ratio
38.3	36.0	1.1

Source: 2009 National Healthcare Quality Report. Reprinted with permission from CDC.gov. (HHS and AHRQ, 2009)

Table 7-10. Percent of children age 2-17 for whom a doctor or other health provider ever gave advice about eating healthy, United States, 2006

Non-Hispanic Black	Non-Hispanic White	Non-Hispanic Black/ Non-Hispanic White Ratio
57.5	56.8	1.0

Source: 2009 National Healthcare Quality Report. Reprinted with permission from CDC.gov. (HHS and AHRQ, 2009)

Not surprisingly, the percentage of overweight people who are told they are overweight appears to increase by age. This means that a doctor is more likely to tell a parent of an 8-year-old that the child is overweight, than the doctor is to tell the parent that a 3-year-old is overweight.

- Are clinicians shirking the subject among younger patients, hoping that growth curves will stabilize?
- Are clinicians now understanding more about the health consequences of early intervention for obesity?
- Policies to monitor younger and counsel younger patients will surely be needed to equalize education and intervention for all groups of all ages (HHS and AHRQ, 2009).

> **NOTE:** Until recently, doctors were not overly concerned about childhood obesity, which is why children and parents were far less likely to be given any help with regards to nutrition or fitness by a doctor or nurse.
> Even now, an obese adult is far more likely than a child to a) be told he or she is overweight and the likely health consequences if nothing is done about it and b) be given counseling regarding nutrition and/or fitness. With the obesity epidemic, this needs to change, and quickly.

Summary

This guide highlights the fact that childhood obesity has increased dramatically over the past three decades. Statistics demonstrate that *all* sectors of the population have their share of obesity rates, and these rates are increasing across all races, age groups, and even socioeconomic groups. But unless we also understand specific trends, we won't know what can be done about it.

This is why nurses *must* help to identify the children at risk of obesity, and also need to help children (and parents) understand that obesity doesn't just happen overnight. With few exceptions, children become obese because of two reasons – they eat too much (or eat too many foods that are high in fat and salt, but are low in fiber, vitamins and minerals, that don't fill them) and exercise too little. Nurses understand the relationship between obesity and the child's nutrition and fitness levels. This is why we're in a unique position to help children, and we must use our position accordingly in order to be the child/patient's best advocate.

In addition, we nurses need to be aware of two significant eating disorders that typically affect teenage girls and young women – anorexia nervosa and bulimia nervosa. We must keep in mind that undereating is every bit as dangerous as overeating – in fact, undereating is potentially far more dangerous as it likely to impair growth in the developing child or young adult. And we must also realize that when someone purges the food he or she has already eaten, many vital nutrients are lost in the process, which may impair growth.

References

Cadman, D., Walter, S.D., Chambers, L.W., Ferguson, R., Szatmari, P., Johnson, N., McNamee, J. (1988). Predicting problems in school performance from preschool health, developmental and behavioural assessments. *CMAJ*. Jul 1;139(1):31-6.

Harbaugh, B.L., Kolbo, J.R., Molaison, E.F., Hudson, G.M, Zhan, L., Wells, D. (2011). Obesity and Overweight Prevalence among a Mississippi Low-Income Preschool Population: A Five-Year Comparison. *ISRN Nurs*.2011:270464. Epub 2011 Sep 18.

Lee, J.M., Appugliese, D., Kaciroti, N., Corwyn, R.F., Bradley, R.H., Lumeng, J.C .(2007). Weight status in young girls and the onset of puberty. *Pediatrics*. Mar;119(3):e624-30.

Lee, J.M., Appugliese, D., Kaciroti, N., Corwyn, R.F., Bradley, R.H., Lumeng, J.C. (2007). Weight status in young girls and the onset of puberty. *Pediatrics*. Mar;119(3):e624-30.

Lee, J.M., Kaciroti, N., Appugliese, D., Corwyn, R.F., Bradley, R.H., Lumeng, J.C. (2010). Body mass index and timing of pubertal initiation in boys. *Archives of Pediatric Adolescent Medicine*. Feb;164(2):139-44.

Magnusson, K.T. (2011). *International Journal of Behavior*. Nutrition Physical Act, 138.

National Center for Health Statistics, (2010) Health Obesity: Percentage of Children ages 6-17 who are obese by race and hispanic origin, age and gender. Selected years 1976-2008. National Health and Nutrition Examination Survey. Retrieved 04/10/12 from http://www.childstats.gov/americaschildren/tables/health7.asp

Tanner, J.M. (1962) *Growth At Adolescence*. Oxford: Blackwell Scientific Publications.

United States Department of Agriculture, (USDA), 2012. Choose My Plate. Retrieved 12/10/11 from www.choosemyplate.gov

United States Department of Health and Human Services (HHS) and Agency for Healthcare Research and Quality (AHRQ) (2009). National Healthcare Disparities Report. Retrieved 01/16/12 from http://www.ahrq.gov/qual/qrdr09/index.html

United States Department of Health and Human Services (HHS) and Agency for Healthcare Research and Quality (AHRQ) (2009). National Healthcare Disparities Report. Retrieved 01/16/12 from http://www.ahrq.gov/qual/qrdr09/6_maternalchildhealth/T6_4_4-1.htm

United States Department of Health and Human Services (HHS) and US Department of Agriculture (USDA) (2010). Secretary's Advisory Committee on National Health Promotion and Disease Prevention Objectives for 2020 July 26, 2010. Retrieved 02/24/12 from http://healthypeople.gov/2020/about/advisory/SocietalDeterminantsHealth.pdf

Zampollo, F., Kniffin, K. M., Wansink, B. and Shimizu, M. (2012), Add Color and Variety to Children's Plates! *Acta Paediatrica*, 101: 61–66 Retrieved on 04/13/12 at http://foodpsychology.cornell.edu/outreach/child-plate.html

Zhang, Q., and Wang, Y. (2004). Trends in the association between obesity and socioeconomic status in U.S. adults: 1971 to 2000. *Obesity Research Journal*. Retrieved 03/12/12 from http://www.ncbi.nlm.nih.gov/pubmed/15536226

Chapter 8
Adolescence, Health & Obesity

"The physical and emotional health of an entire generation and the economic health and security of our nation is at stake."

— First Lady Michelle Obama at the Let's Move! launch
February 9, 2010

This chapter focuses on health promotion and obesity prevention among adolescents. But before understanding the issue at hand, we must emphasize how adolescence is a formative time in our children's lives that can challenge *all* children, be they overweight, obese, underweight, or of healthy weight. As adolescents struggle with issues of self-identity, independence, and a new body transformation, health literacy and health promotion are of utmost importance. Before understanding how to educate adolescents to prevent obesity and promote health, nurses must first have a basic knowledge of the overall health needs of this age group.

In an attempt to better understand the health-related behaviors of typical adolescent youth, the Centers for Disease Control and Prevention (CDC) conducts a Youth Risk Behaviors Surveillance Survey (YRBSS) to monitor six behaviors that contribute to the leading causes of morbidity and mortality (Eaton et al., 2012).

Among teenagers, the six categories included in YRBSS are the following:

1. Injury and violence-related behavior
2. Tobacco use
3. Alcohol and other drug use
4. Sexual behaviors leading to unintentional pregnancy, human immunodeficiency virus (HIV), and sexually transmitted diseases (STDs)
5. Unhealthy dietary behaviors
6. Physical inactivity

While nutrition and fitness seem to make an honorable mention as the fifth and sixth categories, they have not been among the top health-risk behaviors. Results from the 2011 YRBSS gathered information from teenagers in grades 9 to 12 from 43 states and 21 urban school districts. Rates of various behaviors above were gathered and found that nearly half of the students had sexual encounters, 38.7% had consumed alcohol, and 32.8% had been in a fight, and 7.8% had attempted suicide (Eaton et al., 2012). In the same study, high school student behaviors regarding nutrition and fitness demonstrated that 4.8% of students had not eaten fruit (or consumed 100% fruit juice), 5.7% had not eaten vegetables, and 31% had played video games for three hours or more a day over the last 7 days. Although YRBSS attempts to include nutrition and physical activity behaviors, this has little impact on *how* or *why* intervention is needed to reduce obesity among adolescents. The severe impact of obesity and subsequent morbidity must be explained.

We presume that, as more and more children and teenagers struggle with obesity and related health conditions, more and more research will demonstrate how obesity does, in fact, affect the overall health of adolescents and their future global health. An Australian study by Wake et. al. (2012) was the first (and was published today, June 12, 2012) to study obese, overweight, under weight and normal weight children ages 2 to 18 to determine how the *deviation from normal weight affects morbidity across different age groups*. Global health, psychological, and physical health were compared using categories of BMI and parent report, and comorbidities were compared. Measures of poorer health varied less among the younger children (age 2-5), but with older children (starting at age 6 or 7), rise in BMI (and obesity) correlated with poorer global health, asthma, and sleep problems. Additionally, the children of normal weight tended to have the best psychosocial and mental health. Because physiological, anatomical, emotional, and psychosocial changes occur for all adolescents, and *obesity is associated with poorer overall adolescent health*, nurses must strategically teach the importance of child and adolescent health.

Although the hope is that, by teenage years, individuals will have a basic knowledge of health, generally speaking, teenagers seldom receive more health education than basic sex education during their early teen years. With the rise in obesity prevalence across the lifespan, we must focus on early identification of overweight and obese children, and promote developmentally-appropriate strategies to incorporate into their needed health education, in an effort to prevent future weight problems.

The HERO Guide to Health

> **Chapter 8 Objectives:**
> 1. Explain the prevalence of obesity during adolescence
> 2. Outline social, physical, and mental health issues related to obesity and adolescents
> 3. Compare gender differences during adolescent growth and development

The tripling of childhood obesity rates has led to more obesity among adolescents than ever before. The obesity epidemic among teenagers is relatively new, as the highest risk of obesity has typically been among the middle-aged population. Now, we see not only higher rates of obesity, but also significant health disparities among boys and girls, and people of different races (white and black) (CDC, 2010).

Look at the following statistics to see not only how significant the rates of overweight and obese high school students are, but also to understand the gender differences.

Adolescents

Table 8-1. Percentage of Overweight High School Students

	Black	White	Black / White Ratio
Girls	23.3	13.2	1.8
Boys	18.7	13.9	1.3

Source: CDC, 2010. Youth Risk Behavior Surveillance - United States, 2009. Table 90. Reprinted with permission from the CDC.gov.

Table 8-2. Percentage of Obese High School Students

	Black	White	Black / White Ratio
Girls	12.6	6.2	2.0
Boys	17.5	13.8	1.3

Source: CDC, 2010. Youth Risk Behavior Surveillance - United States, 2009. Table 90. Reprinted with permission from the CDC.gov.

8: Adolescence, Health & Obesity

Understanding how significant the gender differences are related to the risk of obesity can help to strategically plan programming for the highest risk adolescents. We know that girls and boys are not the same in many ways, but this demonstrates the significantly higher rates of overweight girls over overweight boys. Nurses must learn how to promote health specifically for boys, and specifically for girls, as their unique group needs are so different in many ways. Physically, anatomically, emotionally and socially, boys and girls must have health promotion geared towards the specific changes they undergo by gender. Beyond segregating boys and girls for a sex education on use of condoms and use of tampons respectively, health education must take into consideration their individual and unique health habits and risk of obesity and comorbidities.

Between the ages of eleven and eighteen, the body experiences a plethora of changes, both internally and externally. It can be a difficult time for many, with unprecedented changes coming rapidly and without warning. It is imperative that, during this time of growth, health issues are addressed with full transparency. Discussion about bodily changes, genital growth, breast growth, hair, and body odor should all be discussed. Just as nurses must first understand the normal physical assessment before understanding what is atypical, so must boys and girls understand normal growth and development during adolescence.

Because of the many physical changes that occur over a short period of time, along with the many psychosocial issues, adolescence is a crucial time for appropriate healthy habits to be learned and encouraged. Nurses can help adolescents and their parents to understand the following:

- Obesity is not a natural course of development or growth during puberty.
- Height/Weight/BMI are useful tools for monitoring growth.
- Nutrition and fitness should be a family endeavor (teens will be less likely to eat fresh fruit if they have never seen it eaten at home).
- Teenagers (despite their independent streak) still look to adults for modeling healthy behaviors – a father jogging with a son can encourage exercise, while bonding as well.
- Girls are beginning to menstruate at younger ages over the past few decades.
- Girls are growing breasts earlier, but obesity is contributing to breast growth.
- Both boys and girls need acceptance and openness about their bodily changes.
- Boys are socially expected to be athletic and strong. Encouraging overweight boys to participate and continue in athletics, when they feel slower and less successful, is a challenge that takes time to overcome, both physically and emotionally.

Puberty and gender differences between boys and girls are significant even when children are of normal weight. With the compounding challenges of obesity among male and female teenagers, the need for health promotion and guidance is crucial. Illness prevention and health promotion should become the hallmarks of pediatric practice and continue throughout adolescence until age eighteen, when teens graduate from a pediatric practice.

Nurses must focus not only on the growth chart and numbers, but also on the consequences and long-term educational needs of the teen to adopt healthy weight patterns as well. The trend of continued obesity from childhood until adulthood poses an unprecedented burden in terms of adolescent chronic health issues, which is one reason why we wish to reverse this trend.

As children grow older and face the somewhat daunting age of adolescence, obesity can continue or *develop* due to poor dietary choices, and be exacerbated by inactivity. Whether or not a child is *diagnosed* as having a weight or metabolic condition, there should be an awareness of obesity prevention and possible strategies. Obesity is difficult to hide, though too easy to ignore. Parents should be made aware of the long-term effects of obesity (Gyovai et al, 2003).

This can be difficult, because the teenage body is a unique construct, floating between childhood and adulthood. The body, at this developmental stage, transforms dramatically both internally and externally. Many facets of puberty and body change are easily camouflaged, which is why parents – and teenagers – can get so confused.

In addition, understanding the adolescent's sexual stage of maturity is also significant because his or her caloric needs and metabolism are in flux during the time of changes and "growth spurts." Consider that a prepubescent teen (who is not yet sexually mature) does not need the added calories that his friend of the same age who has gone through puberty will. That prepubescent teen will also have less muscle mass than his pubertal friend, and will gain more fat if the calories consumed are greater than calories burned – which is easy to do if both teens "hang out" and eat exactly the same food, even though they don't have the exact, same caloric needs. Food choices contribute significantly to adolescent obesity (Wardle et al, 2001).

One important difference between adolescent boys and girls is the nature of sports. Boys are encouraged to play sports throughout this period of change, but girls may lose interest in physically demanding sports and activities, opting for other social activities. The reason for this is because girls have a tendency to become less active during adolescence; this seems to be because inactive girls are accepted as "the norm." During this time, young girls need to be positively influenced into healthy, active living and should be just as encouraged to partake in some type of sport or regular physical activity as the boys are. Young girls from racial minorities have heightened incidences of obesity even at an early age (Wadden et al, 1990).

Some family behavior also seems to be at work, which is why nurses have to keep the parents in mind when activities are encouraged. The fact is, girls need some kind of regular exercise. This needs to be conveyed to the parents, especially if they don't seem to think there's anything wrong with their previously active adolescent girl suddenly becoming inactive because of societal pressure. Nurses must fight the mistaken belief that exercise "isn't necessary" for an adolescent girl.

A combination of hormonal increases and significant physical transformation makes adolescence a critical time for instilling and reinforcing healthy behavior. Puberty is challenging for the teenagers *and* their parents, though in different ways. The nurse should be a guiding force and sounding board for both. As a medical professional, it is essential to understand that, when children commence puberty, it is often just as much of an adjustment for the parent or guardian as it is for the adolescent. The parents' perceived lack of influence or control challenges an already fragile time for the teen, and the teens' desire for independence and social acceptance by peers guides the teens' choices. Nurses can help both parents and teenagers understand the health needs in context of the psychosocial changes at play during this time of metamorphosis.

During puberty, the concept of body image begins to emerge. As peer pressure becomes more significant, girls in particular become more concerned about how they look, what they wear, with extreme pressure to "fit in" to the "right" social group. Having the right look, the right clothes, and listening to the right music are all social side effects of being a teenager.

While you cannot *fully* control these social parameters of adolescence, you *can* still make a positive impact by continuing to give constructive health advice and education. This is important, especially for overweight or obese teens. For example, overweight teenage girls often suffer from low self-esteem and low confidence; if you give them a strategy that will help them to lose weight in a healthy way, they will be likely to appreciate it.

Granted, talking to your patient about his or her weight is not an easy task. With the teenage body changing so quickly, it is important for these young adults to harness and understand the external and intrinsic benefits of a healthy lifestyle.

Women and the concept of "body image" almost becomes synonymous after the age of thirteen, with a large proportion of articles published on female puberty changes and the emergence of the concept of body image. While teenage girls (and women) are often targeted, their male counterparts are *just* as susceptible to body image issues. Eating disorders, such as bulimia and anorexia nervosa, are potentially lifelong and tortuous disorders that can affect both males and females (as we've already seen in Chapter 6). With the rise in obesity, we must not forget how the push to reduce weight can spiral into an eating disorder.

Throughout puberty, the body shape of young boys changes dramatically with periodic growth spurts, hair growth, hormonal increases and a robust appetite. As boys go through puberty, they are less willing by nature to discuss these changes than girls of a similar age. Boys also have a tendency to remain stoic and nonchalant on the outside.

In the midst of such constant change, teenagers have a tendency not to listen to advice from their parents or caregivers. They are usually more responsive to people outside of the family – which is why you, the nurse, need to openly discuss these changes and why they are happening with even the most monosyllabic adolescent male.

It is imperative that the benefits of good, balanced nutrition and exercise are conveyed. While healthy behaviors cannot control or abate every aspect of puberty, knowing and understanding why some choices are better than others can lead to greater self-confidence, with teenagers making the right choices independently and consistently. For example, understanding the insecurities of the individual teenager can help guide how to approach him/her. For instance, an overweight boy might subtly describe body insecurities, and therefore wish to build muscle to replace fat. As nurse, you can initiate a discussion about eating high protein foods to build muscle, in conjunction with aerobic activity. A plan should include a sensible goal that the teenager understands in his own social context. Likewise, a thin teenage boy might be motivated to increase intake of healthier fats (like those in milk, cheese, nuts, and avocado) to bulk up while still eating nutritiously. And his exercise goals might include more muscle-building strength activities. Adolescents must learn and become accustomed to eating and enjoying healthy foods in moderate amounts and, similarly, take part in regular exercise to maintain a desirable and healthy weight range.

For teenagers and parents, obesity is an exceptionally sensitive subject and it is important *not to focus solely on weight loss or body image*. Emphasizing positive attributes and characteristics, and providing a stable environment for teenagers is just as important.

The family *as a whole* needs to make a concerted effort to make smarter choices, as it's easier for people to lose weight if everyone in the family eats the same way. While some in the family may not like this, they need to understand that obesity frequently becomes a lifelong issue; a temporary sacrifice for others may make the difference between a healthy, active life for the overweight or obese teen – or one filled with medical problems, stress, and anxiety (Gyovai et al, 2003).

A family "weight loss" (or weight maintenance) strategy may prove to the best way to go in another sense, as American society as a whole continues to become more sedentary. Ultimately, it will take the strong efforts of many people of all ages to reverse this trend.

There is a reason for it, albeit one that brings to mind the "law of unintended consequences." Because we've had an unprecedented amount of technological change in the past few hundred years, sedentary lifestyles now predominate worldwide. This is because these same advances reduce the need for day-to-day interaction and associated physical activity.

To put it another way: if all of us were suddenly transported to the year 1800, we would have to exercise a whole lot more because it would be *necessary*. If we lived back then, we might have to walk *miles* to go to the store, to go to work, or to visit friends. Even older people today can remember walking more than our children now do – and this was not in the year 1800. We might have to ride a horse to go somewhere that's not within walking distance (horseback riding, while easier on the body in some senses than long-distance walking, is still exercise).

Continuing on, we would also have to do our laundry, which back then involved brushes, big tubs, and a great deal of hard, time-consuming labor. And we'd have to cook most (if not all) of our own food unless we lived in a major municipality – which also would take effort (much more effort than simply popping a prepackaged dinner into the microwave). All of these activities would use *many* more calories than today's far more sedentary lifestyle, which might be why obesity used to be an unusual occurrence.

Here are a few of the contemporary factors that contribute to the inactivity of teenagers and adults:

- Teenagers are less likely to walk or ride a bicycle to or from school, with many being driven or taking public transportation.
- After school programs tend to be sedentary activities which focus on study rather than a balance of fresh air, study, and physical activity.
- Television accounts for a significant amount of time after school; in many households, both parents work, so it can be difficult to monitor and restrict viewing times.
- Teens go to the library less, as the World Wide Web has reduced the need to leave home to look for resources.
- Video and computer games are prevalent and portable; children have access to them almost anywhere.
- Fast food is available almost everywhere, at any time, and families eat out more than ever before.
- Cheap snacks are sugar laden, carbohydrate and fat dense, and readily available.
- Portion sizes have almost doubled.

Obesity is a sensitive issue at any stage of life, but obesity in adolescents comes with a heightened sense of *defensiveness*. This means any form of intervention and/or treatment has the capacity to be both controversial and difficult.

The evaluation of teenage patients is frequently conducted with a parent or guardian in the room. But we know that teenagers are more likely to give open and honest answers if we speak with them privately, without an adult being present. While the parent may not be used to this, explain to them that it will just be a few, routine questions and anything discussed with the adolescent will be similarly discussed with the parent or guardian later. Depending on the parent's relationship with the minor, the child might speak more freely with a nurse. While the entire assessment is unlikely to be without the parent or guardian, the information you gather (if you can establish some privacy) will allow for a more informed analysis of the possible causative factors of obesity.

If you are unable to assess the teenager independently, make sure that your questions are directed toward the individual and encourage him to answer the questions honestly. In some instances, parents will interject and attempt to answer questions on behalf of the patient. Again, obesity is an exceptionally sensitive issue and, sometimes, people – especially parents, as they may feel this is a slight against their parenting skills – may interpret the assessment as a blame-seeking mission. This mindset needs to be allayed in order to conduct a factual assessment.

To highlight health history issues, the following topics should be discussed:

Food preferences: We need to know what types of food are consumed by the individual (including the sizes of the portions). Understanding what the rest of the family eats, along with the readily available choices and the attitude toward food, is imperative. If you don't know the current (and historical) attitude toward food, this will actively hinder the nutrition education process.

Questions to ask regarding food preferences include (but are not limited to):
- Any food allergies or aversions?
- How much grilled lean meat is consumed?
- What type of bread is eaten in the household?
- What is considered a standard breakfast?
- Are fresh fruits and vegetables readily available in the household?
- How often does the family or individual eat out? (The follow-up questions would be, When they do eat out, where do they eat?)
- Does the individual take lunch to school or purchase it there? (The follow-up, providing the teen purchases lunch at school, would be, "When lunch is purchased, what types of choices do you typically make?")
- On an average day, how much water, juice and soda do they consume? (The follow-up: "Do you drink regular, or diet, soda?")
- What types of snacks are available in the household? Is there a significant amount of processed sugary food?
- Are dairy and eggs a regular part of the teen's diet?

Physical Activity: Understanding the teenager's current level of **physical activity**, activities they are **interested in**, as well as the **family perspective** on active living and regular exercise are critical to addressing health behaviors. Remember that, for teens, the stigma of a particular activity can be great. Perhaps the individual used to play soccer, but now, in middle school, soccer is only a boy's sport. Some sports do carry a certain stereotype (***Debbie's note:*** *When I was in high school, I remember that students felt that softball players were all lesbians.*), while clearly not evidence-based, might affect the extracurricular choices made. Teens likely will feel uncomfortable voicing such stereotypes, as social stigma is not comfortably discussed with many adults.

Additionally, cultural norms among a demographic might dissuade participation in a certain sport. Some cultures do not value athleticism among women and prefer to have extracurricular activities that are more "gender-specific."

Clearly, adolescence is influenced by many interplaying factors than cannot and will not always be verbalized voluntarily. Yet, certain questions may be broached as to the organized or individual fitness activities of interest to the adolescent. Questions might include:

- Describe any limitations or challenges you have with fitness or physical activities. Any pain? Discomfort?
- How often do you regularly exercise during and after school?
- What types of activities do you enjoy?
- What is the family attitude towards keeping fit and exercising?
- What types of activities do you currently participate in?

Mental Health: One very important question that health care professionals may overlook seems simple, but is actually quite profound. To wit: do you, as the nurse, always remember to ask the patient how he or she feels? Obesity is linked to many concurrent psychological disorders such as depression, sleeping disorders, and eating disorders, and thus psychosocial elements of health must be included.

In addition to a mental health assessment, open-ended questions may include:

- Tell me how you feel about yourself.
- Describe your family and living situation.
- If you could change something about yourself, what would it be?
- How do you feel about school?
- Tell me about your friends/support people.
- How do you feel about being healthy and/or active? (Teens, like adults, may feel they're being healthy, even if they are completely sedentary. That's why nurses need to continue to educate people about fitness throughout life.)

Developmental Growth and Eating Disorders

While the HERO Guide to Health is primarily centered on obesity and its causative factors, it would be remiss of us as healthcare professionals if we did not discuss the prevalent eating disorders that are often an associated byproduct of the psychological effects, peer pressure and social stigmas affiliated with obesity. These disorders include Anorexia nervosa and bulimia.

Anorexia nervosa, a serious disorder in eating behavior, primarily affects young women in their teens and early twenties. This illness is characterized by a pathological fear of weight gain that leads to malnutrition, extreme weight loss, and inadequate caloric intake. Anorexia is found mostly in adolescent women, but anorexia can affect men and women at any age. It is an exceptionally sensitive subject to broach with patients.

Anorexia is characterized by a distorted self-image of being overweight and leads to an indelible **fear of weight gain**, resulting in an almost complete aversion to food. People suffering anorexia continue to deny themselves food when hungry, eat very small portions, and constantly obsess about their weight. Clinically, it might initially be difficult to determine the difference between undereating and a true, clinical presentation of anorexia nervosa, since there is a natural aspect of body image distortion during adolescence. However, anorexia follows a distinctly different course of extreme aversion to food and extreme caloric restriction, causing nutritional deficiency to the point of hospitalization. Unfortunately, with severe enough anorexia, young adults (often teenage girls) must have inpatient re-feeding programs to help them safely increase their caloric intake (Garber et al., 2012).

Bulimia nervosa is an eating disorder often associated with anorexia, sometimes to the point of being interchanged with it. Bulimia should *not* be confused with anorexia; while most commonly affecting women and sharing the underlying causational factors of poor eating habits and body self-image, bulimia has very different characteristics. Bulimia nervosa is defined by the Merriam Webster Dictionary as a serious eating disorder that occurs chiefly in females. It is characterized by compulsive overeating that is usually followed by self-induced vomiting or laxative and/or diuretic abuse, and is often accompanied by guilt and depression. Since people with bulimia often do not appear overtly thin, and may appear to eat "normally" in public, this disorder can be difficult to assess. This hidden and often severe condition can manifest in many ways, and the difficulty overcoming bulimia can be significant.

***

Debbie's story: When I was in nursing school, I had the opportunity to spend a semester abroad with five of my nursing classmates at a nursing school exchange program in Israel. We were all twenty and twenty-one years old and in a new environment (it was a "home away from home" to me, but still within a new course of study), and shared a college dormitory apartment. In the process of getting to know our fellow classmates (as none of us had ever previously lived together), we quickly learned a lot about everyone's various eating, sleeping, and waking behaviors.

Within a few weeks of discovering who bought what, cooked what foods, showered when, and exercised how, we learned something disturbing about one roommate. Slowly (but dramatically), we found that the stashes of cookies, bread, and foods we were all buying were vanishing. The equivalent of a loaf of bread and tub of cream cheese (actually it was ten pita bread pockets and a large tub of hummus) would disappear overnight.

After consideration and some finger pointing, five of us realized that one of us six had a severe eating disorder. This woman was known to go on a daily run for a few hours at a time. She also spent lengthy times in the bathroom, which was quite noticeable as the six of us all shared one, single toilet. That's why it was easy to determine the culprit, but we were at a loss regarding what to do. Most of us were frustrated by the fact that, no matter what we bought, this other woman kept eating it – and at first, our focus was on the actual food expenses rather than this other woman's health, even though we were nursing students.

We soon realized we had to somehow address this situation. I approached the girl sensitively, without accusation, and discussed what I had noticed. I told her that I was concerned for her due to how much she was working out, and that I often heard her awake at night. She denied her nighttime binges and appeared to truly not remember eating overnight, which concerned me even more. I encouraged the others to offer support rather than frustration, recognizing that this young woman clearly had significant issues with bulimia.

Within a few days of our conversation, our semester abroad was abruptly aborted due to political instability in Israel, and we were sent home to Philadelphia. I remained in contact with my classmate and remember sitting with her to discuss her eating. I knew that she was engaged to a psychology graduate student, and I hoped she would reveal her struggle to him. She, of course, was afraid she would lose him.

For various reasons, despite my attempt to reach out to her and refer her to student health, she stopped talking to me. I think she was embarrassed of what had previously been her dark secret.

***

Both anorexia and bulimia are severe psychological disorders stemming from low self-esteem and an unhealthy obsession with body image and being thin. While the patient might actually be underweight, he or she will view himself or herself as overweight and unattractive, resulting in an unyielding desire to lose weight.

Despite the overarching similarities between bulimia and anorexia, there is a different clinical course, both physically and emotionally. While those suffering from anorexia eat minimal portions and infrequently, bulimics often gorge on food and overeat in an attempt to disguise their obsession. Bulimics will then purge to remove the food from their body, often consumed with guilt and self-loathing. The profound psychological and physical affects of both anorexia and bulimia are all-consuming (Bachrach et al, 1990).

It is imperative for healthcare professionals to be aware of the precursors and symptoms of these disorders. The subject of being too thin is rarely broached, with the signs of anorexia often dismissed as growth spurts and body transformations associated with puberty. Both of these serious disorders require medical intervention as soon as they are recognized (Rosen, 2010).

Finally, we would be remiss if we didn't discuss the current use of medical treatments for obesity, including obesity in adolescence. These types of treatments often contain a heavy push for surgical procedures, such as gastric bypass surgery. While a quick treatment might seem easiest, patients must understand there is no "quick fix" or magic pill. Even after surgery, the very same lifestyle changes must be applied, with dedication and perseverance, or the weight loss will be unlikely to be sustained.

The best option, especially when regarding adolescents, is to make slow changes that will be likely to be sustained. As the nurse, remember always to tell adolescents that any positive change, no matter how small, is a heroic action (one which the HERO program definitely approves of!). Praise that teenager, because he (or she) has taken the initiative to learn what works for him, or her.

Down the line, all of these "slow fixes" are what will lead to real, sustained results. If we are able to teach teens (and their parents) how to eat well and exercise to tolerance, the United States will be a far more healthy, and happy, place.

Summary

Adolescence is a tumultuous time of physical growth coupled with mental advancement and should be treated with a certain level of discretion. Equally important is honesty, a vital component when addressing the root causes of obesity, along with the serious illnesses that obesity may affect, or be a precursor to, later in life.

Obesity in adolescents is often a multi-tiered issue. It is important to ask questions that will give you some understanding of how healthy the current home life is and where changes can be incorporated to facilitate healthier living; these questions fall into four main categories:

1. Physical health.
2. Mental health.
3. Fitness education, including current level of activities and how the teen in question feels about fitness.
4. Nutritional education, including questions about how the teen's parents and family tends to eat, what food likes and dislikes the teen specifically has, and whether the family (or teen) eats out a great deal.

Parents are just as likely to benefit from health education as their adolescent children. They, too, need to understand how they can assist in facilitating change day-to-day in order to increase healthy behaviors and choices (Wadden, 1990).

Adolescents and their families must realize that they can, indeed, make positive, informed lifestyle changes and choices. Whether treating the adolescent individually or the family as a unit, the nurse can help them make these positive choices.

It is imperative for all involved to understand that any changes, no matter how slight, are *heroic*. This is because change, at any level, is difficult, so when a positive transformation is made (no matter what variation), be positive about it!

References

Anorexia Nervosa. 2012. In *Merriam-Webster*.com. Retrieved 03/08/12 from http://www.merriamwebster.com/dictionary/anorexia

Bachrach, L.K., Guido, D., Katzman, D., Litt, I., and Marcus, R. (1990) Decreased Bone Density in Adolescent Girls With Anorexia Nervosa. *Pediatrics by the American Academy of Pediatrics*. Vol. 86 No. 3 September 1, 1990.

Centers for Disease Control (CDC), 2010 Youth Risk Behavior Surveillance - United States, 2009. Table 90. Retrieved on 11/22/11 from: http://www.cdc.gov/mmwr/pdf/ss/ss5905.pdf. Reprinted with the permission of CDC.

Eaton, D.K., Kann, L., Kinchen, S., Shanklin, S., Flint, K.H., Hawkins, J., Harris, W.A., Lowry, R., McManus, T., Chyen, D., Whittle, L., Lim, C., Wechsler, H. (2012). MMWR Surveill Summ. 2012 Jun 8;61(4):1-162. Youth risk behavior surveillance - United States, 2011. 1Division of Adolescent and School Health, National Center for HIV/AIDS, Viral Hepatitis, STD, and TB Prevention, CDC.

Garber, A.K., Michihata, N., Hetnal, K., Shafer, M.A., Moscicki, A.B. *Journal of Adolescent Health* (2012). A prospective examination of weight gain in hospitalized adolescents with anorexia nervosa on a recommended refeeding protocol. Jan;50(1):24-9. E-publication on 2011 Aug 26. Retrieved on 02/27/12 at http://www.ncbi.nlm.nih.gov/pubmed/22188830

Gyovai, V., Gonzales, J., Ferran, K., and Wolff, C. (2003). Family Dietary and Activity Behaviors Associated with Overweight Risk Among Low-income Preschool Age Children. *Californian Journal of Health Promotion*. 2003, Volume 1, Issue 2, Pages 66-77.

Rosen, D. (2010). Identification and Management of Eating Disorders in Children and Adolescents. *Pediatrics Journal by the American Academy of Pediatrics*. Vol. 126 No. 6 December 1, 2010 pp. 1240 -1253 (doi: 10.1542/peds.2010-2821).

Wadden, T., Stunkard, A., Rich, L., Rubin, C., and Sweidel, G. (1990). Obesity in Black Adolescent Girls: A Controlled Clinical Trial of Treatment by Diet, Behavior

Modification, and Parental Support. *Pediatrics Journal by the American Academy of Pediatrics.* Vol. 85 No. 3 March 1, 1990 P 345-353.

Wake, M., Clifford, S.A., Patton, G.C., Waters, E., Williams, J., Canterford, L., Carlin, J.B. (2012). Morbidity patterns among the underweight, overweight and obese between 2 and 18 years: population-based cross-sectional analyses. *International Journal of Obesity (Lond)*. Jun 12. doi: 10.1038/ijo.2012.86. [Epub ahead of print]. Retrieved on 06/12/12 at http://www.ncbi.nlm.nih.gov/pubmed/22689070

Wardle, J., Guthrie, C., Sanderson, S., Birch, L., and Plomin, R. (2001). Food and activity preferences in children of lean and obese parents. *International Journal of Obesity* July 25 (7): 971-7.

Chapter 9
Adult Health & Obesity

"Healthy citizens are the greatest asset any country can have."
— Winston Churchill

In chapters 7 and 8, we explored the growth and development of children and adolescents, and how the childhood obesity epidemic challenges our population at younger ages. Throughout this guide, we continue to emphasize how obesity has been attributed to earlier onset and prevalence of many chronic conditions. This chapter focuses on the need to properly assess the status of our adult patient in the context of obesity. To focus on health promotion, obesity prevention, and care of adult patients and individuals, we pay close attention to two key objectives:

> Chapter 9 Objectives:
> 1. Explain Metabolic Syndrome as a cluster of cardio-metabolic risk factors
> 2. Justify the importance of assessing the adult patient's medical health status as it relates to obesity, nutrition, and exercise

This chapter focuses on adulthood, obesity, and health issues (including cancer) during early and middle adulthood. Depending upon the culture, context, and demographics, adulthood may refer to *biological adulthood* (the attainment of secondary sexual characteristics) or *social adulthood* (the societal or contractual determination of adulthood). In this chapter, we address both biological and social aspects of adulthood in relationship to obesity. We define an adult according to age: between the age of 18 and 64 (and of course beyond 64 as well, though we dedicate a chapter to the care of older adults).

Metabolic Syndrome and Adult Health

Since this portion of the guide serves to help **ASSESS** the health of the adult prior to developing a plan, we must understand all health components related to obesity. Metabolic Syndrome, in a nutshell, helps explain how obesity and health all *interrelate*. Metabolic Syndrome is a conglomeration or clustering of multiple cardio-metabolic risk factors that can lead to heart disease and diabetes (Crist et. al, 2012). There is some controversy as to whether metabolic syndrome is a distinct condition that further raises the heart risks in itself, or merely the sum of all its cluster of cardiac and metabolic components. What differentiates Metabolic Syndrome from other individual conditions is that it appears as a precursor or genetic predisposition to heart disease and diabetes. Metabolic Syndrome can develop insidiously for ten years before diagnosis, thus raising the risk of heart disease and diabetes without the patient even becoming aware of their risks. Central obesity (weight gain around the abdomen or midsection) is a risk factor for Metabolic Syndrome, and thus general obesity awareness can and should educate and promote earlier diagnosis and identification of diabetes, heart disease, high blood pressure and cholesterol, and Metabolic Syndrome.

Metabolic Syndrome, also known as Syndrome X and Insulin Resistance Syndrome, has been known since the 1920s, though it has only been mainstreamed since the 1970s, and was typically a diagnosis of older adults. The incidence of Metabolic Syndrome is 34.3% of adults, ages 20 and greater (Ford & Zhao, 2010). Interestingly, of the 3,461 participants between 2003 and 2006, African Americans had lower rates of Metabolic Syndrome than whites or Mexican Americans, and men had higher rates than women (36.1% compared to 32.4% respectively). Waist circumference measurements were used, and were age- and gender-adjusted. The presence of hypercholesterolemia and hyperinsulinemia had independent positive associations with a diagnosis of Metabolic Syndrome. Also, lower educational status, and fewer leisure time physical activities were associated with higher rates of Metabolic Syndrome.

What diagnoses might be "red flags" for Metabolic Syndrome?
- Diabetes or insulin resistance
- Hypertension
- Central Obesity
- High Cholesterol

All of the above have been common themes throughout this guide. We must understand that, even without central (or midsection) obesity, there can be Metabolic Syndrome. So BMI and weight cannot be a sole identifier of this condition (as we know that no single measurement should diagnose or identify a condition), even though high BMI in itself can elevate the risk of heart disease and diabetes without a specific Metabolic Syndrome diagnosis.

There are a number of organizations that identify criteria to diagnose Metabolic Syndrome. While the goal of this guide is to assess and understand, rather than to diagnose, per se, we will only summarize the criteria to help explain how assessing and managing obesity can reduce the incidence Metabolic Syndrome. Keep in mind that the OBJECTIVE portion of the patient assessment would identify many of these criteria.

Using the World Health Organization criteria from 1999, to have metabolic syndrome, a patient must have:
- **ONE** of the following: diabetes mellitus, *impaired glucose tolerance*, impaired fasting glucose or *insulin resistance*
- AND **TWO** of the following:
  1. Blood pressure: ≥ 140/90 mmHg
  2. *Dyslipidemia*: triglycerides (TG): ≥ 1.695 mmol/L and high-density *lipoprotein* cholesterol (HDL-C) ≤ 0.9 mmol/L (male), ≤ 1.0 mmol/L (female)
  3. Central obesity: waist:hip ratio > 0.90 (male); > 0.85 (female), or body mass index > 30 kg/m2
  4. *Microalbuminuria*: urinary albumin excretion ratio ≥ 20 μg/min or albumin:creatinine ratio ≥ 30 mg/g

Because we see that Metabolic Syndrome involves obesity, high blood pressure, high cholesterol, diabetes, and/or impaired glucose tolerance, we can now appreciate how diet and physical activity are all potential means of improving Metabolic Syndrome as well. Research has demonstrated that an increase in aerobic fitness, with concomitant weight reduction, can decrease the prevalence of metabolic syndrome (Christ et al., 2012). Let us look specifically at heart disease and diabetes, even in isolation, to better understand the trends and health risk factors. When assessing a patient at risk of obesity, or already overweight or obese, it is paramount to assess the risk of heart disease and diabetes.

Heart Disease

As we explored in Chapter 2, heart disease remains the leading cause of death in adults. According to the CDC, the top two ways to *prevent* heart disease are a healthy diet and exercise. Heart disease, of course, is a very broad term that can include many different types of heart disease including: coronary artery disease (CAD), cardiomyopathy (enlarged heart), atrial fibrillation, heart attack, heart valve disease, congenital heart defect, etc. Generally, CAD is the heart disease we refer to when discussing obesity, as CAD is the number one cause of cardiac death in America, and affects 13 million Americans. Obesity increases the risk of CAD, hypertension, high cholesterol, diabetes and many forms of cancer. Thus, for the adult population, educating patients about heart disease must be at the forefront of our health promotion efforts.

Blood Pressure as a Screening Tool for Heart Disease

Patients must understand that, without lifestyle modification as early as possible, perhaps when prehypertension is first discovered, they are likely to develop hypertension and, eventually, heart disease. By explaining the parameters for *prehypertension/at risk* blood pressure (see below), we can help patients understand that *even borderline normal* blood pressures can increase heart disease risk.

Table 9-1. Blood Pressure Levels

Normal	systolic: less than 120 mmHg
	diastolic: less than 80mmHg
At risk (prehypertension)	systolic: 120–139 mmHg
	diastolic: 80–89 mmHg
High	systolic: 140 mmHg or higher
	diastolic: 90 mmHg or higher

Source: Behavioral Risk Factor Surveillance System
Reprinted with permission from the CDC.gov.

The standard of care for improving blood pressure (or to stave off prehypertension) is improved diet and exercise. Yet there are no specific protocols or consistent standards by which physicians promote improved nutrition and exercise. It is more of a cliché catch phrase ... eat better and exercise more. Now what? Many people know they need to do that, but without further education and understanding of how patients can, in fact, successfully improve their medical health, a blood pressure pill seems more likely to succeed. Our mission, as nurses, must be to educate and teach the cause and effect relationship of obesity and medical health, along ways to improve nutrition and fitness.

- Reducing nutritional sodium intake by eating fewer processed/packaged/canned foods
- Substituting herbs and lemon/lime juice – instead of adding salt or salty condiments
- Increasing physical activity to help reduce weight and to exercise the heart

Many people do not recognize *how significant* their food choices are in relationship to obesity and high cholesterol. The nurse can make a tremendous impact through increasing a patient's knowledge of this cause and effect relationship. Help explain the exact diagnoses of the patient, and how each and every diagnosis can be affected by diet and exercise. Verbalizing it to the patient: "You have had high blood pressure since ___ (date) ... you have been on XYZ medication for it, but even increasing activity by X minutes a day ... has been shown to improve blood pressure..." OR – perhaps the patient complains of being on blood pressure diuretics. You can explain how increasing water intake, exercising, and eating more fruits and vegetables can sometimes be effective for blood pressure control – without the use of diuretics. Deciding, along with the physician or nurse practitioner, whether a trial of reducing blood pressure medication (or postponing initiation of medication) can be worthwhile as a long-term health promotion assessment need and plan.

High Cholesterol and Dyslipidemia

Similarly, the assessing for cholesterol management and healthy behaviors is a worthwhile venture for patient and nurse. More and more associations are now being made between atherosclerotic or vascular issues and diabetes. One study from the United Kingdom compared people with early and later onset (before and after age 40) of Type 2 diabetes and compared the lipid profile while on statin medication for high cholesterol (Song & Gray, 2012). Fifty patients with Type 2 diabetes, though without cardiovascular disease, were treated with statins to achieve normal lipid profile. Those with earlier onset of Type 2 diabetes had a greater burden (or effect) of Apolipoprotein B. Younger age and earlier onset of Type 2 diabetes was predictive of higher Apo B. This can be used to emphasize the need for cholesterol screening, especially among those at risk of obesity and/or Type 2 diabetes.

In the OBJECTIVE portion of patient assessment, nurses have the opportunity and need to review and document laboratory findings including LDL, HDL, total cholesterol and triglyceride levels. Pay close attention to lab results, in addition to physical exam findings, and patient eating and fitness habits, as the nurse must incorporate all this information into the patient's health status.

Now, during the **ASSESSMENT**, the nurse should provide even brief nuggets of nutrition and health recommendations for patients to understand. Even if time is short, and the information may seem simple to you, the nurse, we must recognize the tremendous need for and impact of even a few moments of health promotion and education. For example, to reduce the amount of dietary cholesterol, the nurse can take a moment to explain the importance of:

- Choosing lean meats (grilled fish or chicken) instead of a fatty meats (ground beef, sausage, veal, and deep fried meats)
- Eating high fiber foods (beans, leafy greens, whole grains)
- Choosing low fat milk and low fat or part skim cheese
- Increasing aerobic activity to exercise the heart

Diabetes

The above recommendations are also necessary for diabetes teaching. Because of the strong association between obesity, Metabolic Syndrome, and Type 2 diabetes, it is essential that nurses understand the differences between diabetes classifications. In general, in the context of obesity, we refer to Type 2 diabetes, the incidence of which is steadily rising. A study by Koopman et al. (2005) reviewed the National Health and Nutrition Examination Survey (NHANES) from 1999-2000 and the NHANES III from 1988-1994. Researches compared prevalence rates of Type 2 diabetes among adults (aged 20 and older) from both survey periods. The average age of diagnosis of Type 2 diabetes decreased from 52 years old to 46 years old. Although there are many plausible explanations for the decrease in age at diagnosis, obesity certainly can explain this trend (Flegal et al., 2002). In this case, the obesity epidemic has taken a toll on the general care of the adult population. While middle-aged adults a few decades ago were at the start of worrying about Type 2 diabetes, hypertension, and heart disease, adults now often already have lived with chronic conditions for years. Below, we explain the distinct classification of diabetes, as the medical treatment, though similar, may vary.

Summary of Diabetes Classifications

- **Type 1 Diabetes Mellitus (formerly called Juvenile Diabetes):** Usually has onset for the child or adolescent, though onset can be at any age. Type 1 diabetes accounts for 5 to 10% of all diabetes diagnoses. High blood glucose levels due to lack of insulin-producing beta cells cause a dependency on insulin shots. Symptoms such as excessive thirst, frequent urination, blurry vision, extreme fatigue, extreme hunger, and weight loss may be seen. Severe complications can include diabetic *ketoacidosis*, diabetic shock, and severe hypoglycemia (lower than 70mg/dl can cause symptoms). Strict diet management must supplement consistent medical care to reduce complications.

    In the past, it was known that an "apple-shaped" body, versus a "pear-shaped" one could help identify children at risk of diabetes. Today, more research has discovered that, across all ages, the apple-shape versus pear-shape increases the risk of diabetes 6 times, and also increases the risk of heart disease. Thus, in addition to monitoring diet due to insulin and blood sugar balance, monitoring weight among children with diabetes should also be a focus, in order to help reduce obesity and prevent the additional risks associated with increased mid-trunk weight (Savard, 2005).

- **Type 1.5 Diabetes**: Latent Autoimmune Diabetes in Adults (LADA) was discovered in the 1970s and accounts for 10% of all diabetes, being even more common than Type 1 diabetes. LADA appears to be a slow onset Type 1 diabetes seen among adults. One way to differentiate between Type 2 diabetes and LADA, is that adults with LADA tend to have a normal body weight, and often have a family history of Type 1 diabetes or autoimmune disease. LADA tends to require more aggressive treatment with insulin than Type 2 diabetes. Testing pancreatic antibodies can help diagnose LADA, and a specific diagnosis of this form of diabetes is needed for appropriate management of the condition (Johns Hopkins, 2012).

- **Type 2 Diabetes Mellitus** (formerly called Adult Onset Diabetes) is the most commonly diagnosed form of diabetes. The pathophysiology is somewhat different from that of Type 1 Diabetes, though treatment with insulin may also be needed. A combination of *resistance to insulin action* and *inadequate insulin secretion* causes hyperglycemic states. Sometimes controlled by exercise and diet, the person may ultimately require medication and even insulin injections. But because the body still can secrete insulin, the person with Type 2 Diabetes is usually not dependent on insulin. Complications such as *ketoacidosis* can occur, though rarely among patients with Type 2 Diabetes.

    Due to the increase in childhood obesity, Type 2 diabetes is now more commonly diagnosed at younger ages. Signs of diabetes may include polyphagia, polydipsia, polyuria, and even weight loss, ironically, despite the association of Type 2 diabetes with obesity (Khardori, 2012). Again, Dr. Savard described how people are often diagnosed only after significant disease symptoms are discovered, and thus weight and body type should be used as an early diagnosis tool to help diagnose this condition even 10 to 20 years before diabetes might have otherwise been diagnosed (Savard, 2005).

- **Gestational Diabetes Mellitus (GDM)**: can only affect *pregnant women*, and occurs in 5% of pregnancies or 200,000 cases per year (NICHHD, 2008). To diagnose GDM, all pregnant women undergo an oral glucose tolerance test around 24-28 weeks gestation. (If the pregnant woman has a history of diabetes, her diabetes during pregnancy is not considered GDM.) GDM does usually go away shortly after delivery, though the woman should have a follow-up blood glucose test within a few weeks of delivery. Proper eating and exercise should be maintained to balance the glucose and insulin.

Most women with GDM who control their blood sugar and balance diet and exercise deliver healthy babies. But the lifetime risk of developing obesity, abnormal glucose tolerance, and diabetes is increased for both mother and child.

- **Hypoglycemia (low blood sugar)**: defined as a blood sugar lower than 70 mg/dL; this condition is uncommon for people without diabetes. In diabetes, and exacerbated by some diabetes medications and insulin, an impaired response of glucagon (from the pancreas) makes it hard for the body to return blood sugar to normal levels. The low blood sugar can happen rapidly and cause sweating, shakiness, anxiety, and more. Eating or drinking glucose-rich foods right away can help normalize the blood sugar. Without treatment, though, severe hypoglycemia can lead to seizures, coma, and even death (HHS – NDIC, 2012).

   Nurses must realize the complexity of sugar/insulin balance and the influences of both hypo and hyperglycemia. While this guide encourages exercise and balanced nutrition, in the context of diabetes and hypoglycemia, the nurse must fully understand the capacity of the individual in the limitations of their health status. For example, a person with diabetes who takes insulin regularly (let us say for Type 1 or Type 2 diabetes) who suddenly decides to start exercising and lifting weights, would be at risk of becoming hypoglycemic as his energy expenditure (via exercise) would suddenly go up, and he might not have eaten enough or reduced insulin enough to accommodate for the new change.

Nurses must help emphasize the potential severity of complications from diabetes, which can be curbed or prevented with proper nutrition and physical activity. For patients who have been already diagnosed with Type 2 diabetes, nurses must encourage continued monitoring and general care. Just as we monitor blood pressure for heart disease, diabetics must have blood sugar monitoring (both fasting and hemoglobin A1C). Because the outcome and success of treatment for diabetes is largely related to the overall health of the person, nurses *must* be well versed in the general care of a diabetic patient.

According to Healthy People 2020, only 56.8 % of adults aged 18 years and older with *diagnosed* diabetes stated they received formal diabetes education at any time (age adjusted to the year 2000 standard population). Given the significant effect diabetes can have on lifestyle and health status, along with the many complications and morbidities, diabetes education must be a priority (USDA, 2010).

General Care:
- Routine medical exam (history and physical exam)
- Blood Pressure Monitoring
- Self-check blood glucose, if required
- Foot check for diabetic ulcers
- Vision check for diabetic retinopathy
- Routine labs, including fasting blood glucose, Hgb A1C, urine for protein and sugar
- Nutrition Counseling
- Diabetes Education
- Fitness Education

Cancer

We have already discussed cancer and genetics, and their relationship to obesity. But with more and more people at risk of cancer, at risk of diabetes, heart disease, and more, we must understand how to assess and plan for care of adults who may have a history of cancer, are now overweight, and are at risk of other conditions. According to Healthy People 2020, cancer is the leading cause of death, second only to heart disease. In Chapter 2, we discussed the relationship between obesity and cancer, and the many forms of cancer with increased risk associated with obesity. When we assess our patient, and their obesity prevention needs, we must, of course, look at whether they have a history of cancer, are undergoing cancer treatment, or have additional risk factors for cancer.

For a patient who has already been diagnosed with cancer, is in remission, or has a history of cancer, we must assess and recognize how their health might already be impaired, and how their nutrition and fitness needs or ability might be altered. For instance, a patient with a history of colon cancer, with a colostomy bag, might have nutritional absorption issues, might have psychosocial or even physical limitations to fitness activities, etc. Keep in mind the interplay between the many diagnoses and health issues, along with their risk factors; all must be assessed together to successfully plan an individualized health plan.

In addition to the above conditions, the adult population often carries the following comorbidities:

- **Osteoarthritis**
- **Depression**
- **Gastroesophageal Reflux Disease (GERD)**
- **Sleep Apnea**

We have touched on a few elements of the above conditions within the physical exam portion. Of course, *all* of our individual patient's symptoms, diagnoses, psychosocial and behavioral elements, and medication profile must be incorporated into the education and intervention plan. Here, the nurse must lead the way – and **initiate** the conversation about health promotion.

According to the Agency for Healthcare and Research and Quality Survey (2002-2007), there has been slight improvement from 2002 to 2007 regarding percentages of people who receive counseling on healthy eating (48.9% to 51.6% respectively); disparities among populations who receive the counseling remain (AHRQ, 2010). Adults ages 18-44 were least likely to receive advice about healthy eating. And poorer individuals, those with less than a high school education, or Hispanics compared to Whites were less likely to receive counseling on healthy eating and exercise. Strikingly, in 2007 for obese adults, 52.7% of poor compared to 66.6% of high-income adults received counseling on the need for exercise. Survey data from 2005-2008 showed that 65.9% of obese adults age 20 and over reported being told by a doctor or health professional that they were overweight or obese (AHRQ, 2010).

The lack of health education by providers is significant because research shows that engaging in just one lifestyle modification (diet, exercise, smoking cessation, never having been obese) can cut the risk of heart disease, diabetes, and stroke by half (compared to no modification). All four lifestyle modifications can reduce these risks by 78% (AHRQ, 2010). Rather than letting patients like these "fall through the cracks," we should arm ourselves with the knowledge to explain *why* and *how* even small modifications to diet and exercise can improve what otherwise could become a cascade of medical issues, requiring a slew of medicines.

Now is the time and place for the nurse to assess the situation and identify the main health need for the patient. Ask yourself:

- Who is our patient? What are the main health and social issues at hand?
- What are the commonalities of all their symptoms, diagnoses, and health needs?
- What can we teach our patient to take away with them as teaching tools?
- Can nutrition and fitness improve Metabolic Syndrome, high blood pressure, obesity, and high cholesterol? YES, YES, YES!
- How can we promote health behaviors for this *individual* patient?

See Appendix A for a flowchart that can be used to create SOAP notes with a plan. In addition to providing health promotion and discussion of lifestyle modifications, we must provide our patients with concrete plans of care. In the case of high blood pressure, we must emphasize that our patient will require continued blood pressure monitoring, increased fitness, improved nutrition, consistent follow-up. Again, improved eating and fitness is no quick fix, and people genetically predisposed to high blood pressure can eat a vegetarian diet and run marathons and *still* have high blood pressure, so our plan must be highly individualized by fully assessing the patient and his health history, family history, and current health.

Nurses can help develop an appropriate plan to follow-up with routine blood pressure monitoring, while also providing health education and obesity prevention strategies. The U.S. Preventive Services Task Force gives hypertension screening for people aged 18 and older a *Recommendation*, indicating that "there is high certainty that the net benefit is substantial." (The USPSTF, 2007)

As one of the most accessible and inexpensive screening tools, monitoring blood pressure can be an early – and inexpensive – first approach for someone who is overweight or obese. After that, specific strategies for health promotion can and should be addressed.

All of these conditions, even in isolation, can be debilitating to an individual but obesity further increases the risk of such conditions. While heart disease and cancer are the top two causes of mortality and morbidity during the adult years, so many conditions that ail the adult population are linked to obesity, and thus directly or indirectly cause morbidity and mortality in adulthood. In an effort to improve the quality of life for adults, consistent and continued health education *must* be provided. In order to get people to make wise choices independently, health and nutritional education is paramount.

References

Agency for Healthcare Research and Quality (2010). National Healthcare Disparities Report 2010. Retrieved on 07/07/12 at http://www.ahrq.gov/qual/nhdr10/Chap2c.htm

Centers for Disease Control (CDC), 2012, Behavioral Risk Factor Surveillance System. Retrieved 01/14/12 from http://cdc.gov/dhdsp/data_statistics/fact_sheets/fs_bloodpressure.htm

Centers for Disease Control (CDC), 2012, Diabetes and Data Trends. Retrieved 06/07/12 from http://www.cdc.gov/diabetes/statistics

Centers for Disease Control (CDC), 2012, Health and Safety for College Students. Retrieved 06/07/12 from http://cdc.gov/features/collegehealth

Centers for Disease Control (CDC), 2012, Heart Disease Facts and Statistics. Retrieved 05/05/12 from http://www.cdc.gov/heartdisease/statistics.htm

Cheng, S.H., Shih, C.C., Lee, I.H., Hou, Y.W., Chen, K.C., Chen, K.T., Yang, Y.K., Yang, Y.C. (2012). A study on the sleep quality of incoming university students. Psychiatry Research, Feb 17. [Epub ahead of print and retrieved on 02/27/12 at http://www.ncbi.nlm.nih.gov/pubmed/22342120]

Crist, L.A., Champagne, C.M., Corsino, L., Lien, L.F., Zhang, G., & Young, D.R.(2012). Influence of change in aerobic fitness and weight on prevalence of metabolic syndrome. Preventing Chronic Disease. DOI: Retrieved on 07/2/12 at http://www.cdc.gov/pcd/issues/2012/11_0171.htm

Flegal, K.M., Carroll, M.D., Ogden, C.L., Johnson, C.L. Prevalence and trends in obesity among US adults, 1999–2000. JAMA. 2002;288:1723–1727.

Ford, E.S., Li, C., Zhao, G. (2010). Prevalence and correlates of metabolic syndrome based on a harmonious definition among adults in the US. *Journal of Diabetes* 2010;2(3):180-93.

Johns Hopkins Medical Alerts (2012). Is it Type 2 Diabetes or LADA?. Retrieved 02/29/12 from http://www.johnshopkinshealthalerts.com/reports/diabetes/1366-1.html

Khardori, R. (2012). Type 2 Diabetes Mellitus. Medscape. Retrieved 02/13/12 from http://emedicine.medscape.com/article/117853-overview

Koopman, R.J., Mainous, III, A.G., Diaz, V.A., & Geesey, M.A. (2005). Changes in Age at Diagnosis of Type 2 Diabetes Mellitus in the United States, 1988 to 2000. *Annals of Family Medicine*. 2005 January; 3(1): 60–63.doi: 10.1370/afm.214. Retrieved 06/15/12 from http://www.ncbi.nlm.nih.gov/pmc/articles/PMC1466782

National Cancer Institute at the National Institutes of Health (2012). Obesity and Cancer Risk. Retrieved on 04/19/12 at http://www.cancer.gov/cancertopics/factsheet/Risk/obesity

National Institute of Child Health and Human Development. (2008). Gestational Diabetes. Retrieved on 07/05/12 at http://www.nichd.nih.gov/health/topics/gestational_diabetes.cfm

Savard, M. (2005). *Apples & Pears: the Body Shape Solution for Weight Loss and Wellness*. Atria Books, New York.

Song, S.H., Gray, T.A. (2012). Early-onset type 2 diabetes: higher burden of atherogenic apolipoprotein particles during statin treatment. *QJM*. 2012 Jun 28. [Epub ahead of print]. Retrieved on 07/4/12 at http://www.ncbi.nlm.nih.gov/pubmed/22753665

United States Bureau of Labor and Statistics (2012). College Enrollment and Work Activity of 2011 High School Graduates. Retrieved on 07/2/12 at http://www.bls.gov/news.release/hsgec.nr0.htm/

United States Department of Health and Human Services (HHS) and Agency for Healthcare Research and Quality (AHRQ) (2010). National Healthcare Disparities Report. Retrieved 01/16/12 from http://www.ahrq.gov/

United States Department of Health and Human Services (HHS) and Agency for Healthcare Research and Quality (AHRQ) (2012). Retrieved 04/10/12 from http://www.ahrq.gov/qual/nhdr10/Chap2c.htm#lifestyle

United States Department of Health and Human Services (HHS), National Diabetes Information Clearinghouse (NDIC), (2012). Hypoglycemia. Retrieved 02/13/12 from http://diabetes.niddk.nih.gov/dm/pubs/hypoglycemia

United States Department of Health and Human Services (HHS) and US Department of Agriculture (USDA) (2010). Secretary's Advisory Committee on National Health Promotion and Disease Prevention Objectives for 2020 July 26, 2010. Retrieved 02/24/12 from http://healthypeople.gov/2020/about/advisory/SocietalDeterminantsHealth.pdf

U.S. Preventative Task Force (2007). Screening for High Blood Pressure in Adults. Retrieved on 07/06/12 at http://www.uspreventiveservicestaskforce.org/uspstf/uspshype.htm

Chapter 10
Maternal Health & Obesity

The nature of obesity is such that body size and shape may wax and wane throughout the course of our lives. Many of us, even if not overweight now, may have been overweight at one time – maybe even obese. And those of us who are overweight or obese now, likely remember a thinner time. So understanding *all* phases throughout adulthood must be considered in the context of obesity. Thus far, The HERO Guide To Health has discussed many different aspects of health related to obesity among the general adult population. But to thoroughly provide an adult health overview for nurses and the general public alike, we must also include pregnant women.

> Chapter 10 Objectives:
> 1. Identify the appropriate weight gain during pregnancy
> 2. Summarize the risks of underlying obesity in a pregnant woman
> 3. Identify presence of hypertension, diabetes, and obesity during pregnancy
> 4. Determine the nutritional needs of the mother and baby

Despite significant abdominal girth and weight gain during pregnancy, obesity is not a desired or natural progression during pregnancy. Although there is great variability among pregnancies, and weight gain, nurses must understand the difference between appropriate weight gain for the benefit of the fetus, and improper balance of nutrition and exercise, leading to obesity. Because it now seems commonplace to see obese pregnant women (without a prior health history, is would be impossible to know if the weight is pregnancy-related or not) and there is often more "acceptance" of this as a social norm. Thus, whether actively or passively, less effort is made by health practitioners to promote healthier habits and weight during pregnancy.

First, we discuss maternal and infant health. And men, remember that knowledge of infant and female development should be of interest or concern to you as well, even if just in the context of better knowing how to respond to other people's challenges. And given that male nurses, too, must be knowledgeable about the female body, this will act as a refresher, but in the context of obesity.

Maternal and Infant Health

Even before the obesity epidemic, there were always two main issues related to pregnancy: 1) the health of the mother; and 2) the health of the fetus

10: Maternal Health & Obesity

or baby. As we describe throughout this guide, obesity can complicate many facets of health, and can thus make already difficult body transitions even more difficult.

Until the more recent obesity epidemic, prenatal concerns involved whether the mother used alcohol or drugs, smoked, her age at pregnancy, prior health history that might complicate her pregnancy, and such. The health history, similar to a general adult history, would also include how many pregnancies, miscarriages, abortions, and complications such as eclampsia, preeclampsia, gestational diabetes, and gestational hypertension.

Typically, when a woman first discovers she is pregnant, the first course of prenatal care is to schedule a visit with an obstetrician. Using the date of the woman's last menstrual period (LMP), the obstetrician can estimate how many weeks pregnant the woman is, and begin to monitor both the growth of the mother and the fetus. The pregnant woman will have her weight, blood pressure, and certain labs checked routinely. As her due date gets closer, her visits become more frequent, as the potential risks are greater as both mother and baby grow. Just as a child has his growth measured via height, weight, and BMI checks, the pregnant mother has even more frequent measurements, as she is monitored only during the course of her 40 weeks of pregnancy. Remember that, by the time a woman discovers she is pregnant and seeks medical care, she is likely already a few weeks pregnant. At best, a woman has 40 weeks worth of medical monitoring for body changes that are potentially life-altering and sometimes even debilitating (some women become bedridden due to various complications of pregnancy including preeclampsia, eclampsia and more). And, thus, seeking care during this time is critical, even if the woman has no prior obesity or health issues. Some women receive little or no prenatal care.

> **NOTE:** In 1999, I (Debbie) heard of a women who only discovered she was pregnant the day she delivered! While we all have heard of crazy delivery stories, this one takes the cake! (I delivered my son at the very same hospital 4 years later, while standing over the toilet at the Prenatal Evaluation Center, since the nurse did not believe I was having contractions and the obstetrician had not even evaluated me yet). But back to the original story – apparently, the woman was obese (technically, morbidly obese) and had not menstruated in years due to her weight and other factors; she was even too large to feel the baby moving within her. While this certainly is not the norm even among obese pregnant women, it is certainly concerning. Clearly, she was not receiving prenatal care, nor was she reminded, at the least, to improve her habits for the child. And I highly doubt that there was follow-up beyond the delivery to ensure that she had the knowledge and resources to take care of herself and the baby.

Aside from stories like this, for the majority of healthy women, pregnancies progress fairly typically. Women will have variations in weight gain, some fluctuation in blood pressure, and perhaps a few extra tests conducted (certain genetic tests and amniocentesis are not routine, but rather elective, and their added risks must be understood). But, unless the woman needs "high risk" obstetrical care for infertility, or prior health reasons, she will follow a standard course of prenatal visits, with a 6-week follow-up after giving birth.

Emotionally, pregnant women might have mood fluctuations, as hormonal changes occur throughout and after pregnancy (the men need be aware of this – there is a physiological reason for it, to some extent). Morning sickness, food aversions, and food cravings can alter the woman's typical diet. Fatigue, discomfort, and nausea can impair their ability to stay active. Despite these changes, a fairly predictable course usually ensues. And in my (Debbie's) experience (as a mother of two children, and a clinician), seldom is health education fully provided by the obstetrician or nursing staff. Unless a woman takes the initiative to borrow or buy pregnancy-related books, an expectant mother might have little education on the process ahead. How does she learn what to eat, what to do, and how to provide what is needed for herself and the baby? (See information on Women, Infants and Children (WIC) later in this chapter.) And maybe she was already unsure of what to eat before pregnancy.

To understand the effects of obesity on a pregnant woman, we must first know *how high* the risks of pregnancy-related complications are already, even without having the added health burden of obesity. In 2007, 11 per 1,000 pregnant women had chronic hypertension compared to 38 per 1,000 having gestational hypertension, and both were highest among non-Hispanic African women. The rate of any type of diabetes among pregnant women was 44.8 per 1,000 and highest among Hispanic women (HHS, 2010). Now consider the rising rates of hypertension and diabetes across *all* populations, we would expect the pregnancy-related complications to further increase. People must understand how the physiological and anatomical changes that occur during pregnancy can increase the risk of developing gestational hypertension and/or diabetes, and thus nutrition and health before, during, and after pregnancy should be promoted.

Unfortunately, clinical practice often focuses more on acute treatment of low birth-weight infants, rather than on health promotion and prevention for the mothers who carried them. Since 2007, there has been a small decrease in the number of preterm deliveries and low birth weight babies in the U.S., though this seems more related to the birth of multiples (from fertility) and use of cesarean section than related to maternal health. Data from the CDC found that preterm deliveries (before 37 weeks gestation) declined slightly to 12.8% of births and low birth weight deliveries (babies weighing less than 2,500 g) are stable at around 8% (HHS, 2010). This is why focusing on the mothers for prenatal care – not just during their pregnancies – is extremely important. Yet still, these rates are high compared to those in other, less developed countries.

Amnesty International published a scathing report in 2009 highlighting the fact that, from 1987 to 2006, maternal mortality rates in the United States have more than doubled to 13.3 per 100,000 (Amnesty International, 2010). At the same time, the U.S. spends drastically more on healthcare than other countries, and the highest expenses are in maternal-fetal care, but there is a drastically higher rate of maternal complications and death compared to rates in other countries. Maternal death rates are five times higher in the U.S than in Greece, and three times higher than in Spain. In addition to the global disparities, the U.S. continues to have distinct racial disparities for maternal care, and African American women are four times more likely to die of pregnancy-related complications than white women (Amnesty International, 2010).

Relatively little progress has been made in the last 20 years, and the lack of prenatal *and* postnatal care are contributing factors to poorer outcomes for both the mother and baby. Obesity prior to pregnancy *already* increases the risk of diabetes and hypertension, and thus pregnancy-related complications for mother and infant are at increased risk. Regardless of whether the mother is already receiving healthcare for her own needs, those needs are compounded in the face of pregnancy and childbirth. Certainly for low-income mothers, the healthcare system does not always support the added needs, and these mothers may often feel excluded by the current system. Whether the co-payments or costs are daunting and dissuade doctor visits, or there are no accessible and publicly-funded prenatal centers, there is a lack of services rendered for up to 50% of pregnant women. This is why we need to consider the mother who does *not* follow a high-risk lifestyle, but who also does not necessarily follow a healthy path of nutrition and activity.

While research does show the need for healthy eating and exercise during pregnancy, even the current literature lags behind the need to include obesity as a significant topic of focus. A study by Ruchat et al. (2012) clearly shows that women of normal weight who initiated healthy eating and even light to moderate exercise (walking even 3-4 times a week) gained less gestational weight and retained less of the weight after two months post-delivery. Interestingly, the study is a) Canadian – and obesity rates in Canada are lower, medical care is socialized and b) the women were all of normal weight to begin with. We must recognize there would likely be a greater challenge for women who are *already* overweight, and the effects during pregnancy for them need be studied also.

Yes, there are gaps in our healthcare system. Acknowledging this, and moving forward to intervene... what can we do? **Health Education To Reduce Obesity** is a **Must** across all age groups. Accomplishing this remains a challenge, and Heathy People 2020 addresses the issue by striving to increase initiatives for women before they become pregnant (they call this the "life course perspective") (HHS, 2012).

Finally, due to the obesity epidemic, the U.S. will see more and more pregnant women who are already overweight or obese and who have diabetes, hypertension, and/or heart disease. Which raises the following questions:

- How does their health affect their pregnancy?
- How does their health affect the baby's health?

To answer these questions, we must understand how pregnancy affects the body. Nurses know that, in general, during the approximate 40 weeks of gestation, there are physical changes to both the mother and fetus. But what are they, specifically?

Let's look at the three main effects of pregnancy on the human body:
1. **Weight gain**
2. **Increase in blood volume**
3. **Increased nutritional requirements**

> **NOTE:** Any woman who has been pregnant understands that the above three effects of pregnancy hardly scratch the surface of the complex metamorphosis during the 40 weeks or so of pregnancy, much less the resulting changes that may linger for years (or a lifetime) beyond the actual pregnancy.

As this book focuses on obesity and lifestyle changes, we cannot delve into the full scope of pregnancy. Instead, here is a summary of a few target areas:

1. **Weight gain during pregnancy:** You should gain weight gradually during your pregnancy, with most of the weight gained in the last 3 months. Many doctors suggest women gain 1 to 4 pounds (total) during the first three months (or first trimester), then 2 to 4 pounds per month during the 4th to 9th months (second and third trimesters). The total amount of weight you should gain during your pregnancy depends on your weight when you became pregnant; women whose weight was in the healthy range before pregnancy should gain between 25 and 35 pounds while pregnant. The advice is different for those who were overweight or underweight before becoming pregnant.

10: Maternal Health & Obesity

2. **Increase in Blood Volume:** The human body *auto-regulates* to meet the increasing metabolic and hematologic demands of the mother and fetus. Beginning in the 6-8 weeks gestation period, the pregnant woman's blood mass progressively increases to meet this metabolic demand of the mother. Blood plasma volume increases by 30-50%, and red blood cell mass increases by 30-50% (Mayo Clinic, 2012). These changes in blood volume serve two essential purposes:

   - Improve the exchange of respiratory gases, metabolites, and nutrients between the mother and fetus
   - Ensure minimal blood loss during delivery of the baby (fibrinogen and platelets rise, though not above normal limits)

   > **NOTE:** Taking a prenatal vitamin with both iron and folic acid is essential to help maintain normal hemoglobin levels (Ciliberto and Marx, 1998).

   Blood Pressure:

   For a woman with a typical pregnancy who is otherwise healthy, *blood pressure should not increase* compared to their baseline. However, we must recognize that with the increase in young women who are overweight and obese, there will be a far higher percentage of women presenting to their obstetrician with a history of hypertension. Or women who have not been diagnosed with hypertension will assume they will have a normal pregnancy, but find that, with a significant increase in blood volume and stroke volume, they now have increased blood pressure. With this obesity epidemic, more women during childbearing years are developing not only hypertension and pre-eclampsia, but also diabetes (Simmons, 2011).

   Although the babies most commonly are born healthy to mothers with diabetes or hypertension during pregnancy, maternal health does affect the offspring's lifetime risk of heart disease, stroke, and diabetes (NIH, 2008).

   Because of the increased risk of hypertension and diabetes during pregnancy, especially among overweight and obese women, it is imperative that women of childbearing years monitor their weight *before* they become pregnant. Following a healthy lifestyle of proper nutrition and physical activity is essential, not only for the mother and her health before, during, and after pregnancy, but also for the health of the child.

Monitoring the mother before pregnancy for signs of hypertension and diabetes is crucial. But how can we adopt this plan successfully if young women don't get the proper education beforehand? Simple: we can't, which is why we urge women who plan to be mothers to learn more about nutrition. In addition, during adolescent years, young girls need to learn the importance of proper health and nutrition; if they do so, they – and any babies they bear down the line – will be far healthier. (See Chapter 8 for more information regarding adolescence and obesity.)

3. **Increased Nutritional Requirements:** After focusing on the need to monitor overweight women during childbearing years, now we must understand the **increased** nutritional requirements of pregnancy. This is quite confusing to patients, as a young mother might ask, "I was told to eat less, and now I need to eat more?"

    Herein lies the confusion. Eating a healthy diet before and during pregnancy is not so much a matter of *less* or *more* food, but more an issue of *which foods are best*, and how pregnant women can best meet their nutritional requirements This is an extremely opportune time for women to adopt better eating habits overall. This is because they may not have known what to do for themselves, but didn't make much of an effort because it might not have seemed to matter. But because the soon-to-be mother likely wants to do what is best for her child, she may make that effort, if only for her child's sake. In a nutshell, pregnancy is an opportunity to adopt and learn healthier eating habits.

WIC and Other Helpful Programs

What nutritional services are there outside of a physician's office? One federal program for which new mothers may qualify, called Women, Infant, and Children (also known as *WIC*), is available through the USDA and the Food and Nutrition Service. WIC is probably the best resource for nutrition of mothers, infants, and children until age 5. WIC, focused on low-income mothers and children, along with those at nutritional risk, provides not only financial assistance for purchasing healthy food for the mother and child, but also educational and nutritional services.

There are certain criteria that women and children must meet to be eligible to participate in the WIC program. Though nearly 7 billion dollars was appropriated by Congress for the 2010 WIC Program, not every person receives benefits ("Eligibility Requirements.") (FNS, 2012). Physicians, nurses, dieticians, and other practitioners assess the patient for eligibility, and the priority for available participation follows the list below from highest to lowest priority:

First are **pregnant women, breastfeeding women, and infants** determined to be at nutritional risk because of nutrition-related medical conditions.

Second are **infants up to 6 months of age** whose mothers participated in WIC or could have participated and had a medical problem.

Third are **children at nutritional risk** because of **nutrition-related medical problems**.

Fourth are **pregnant or breastfeeding women and infants** at nutritional risk because of **inadequate dietary patterns**.

Fifth are **children at nutritional risk** because of **inadequate dietary patterns**.

Sixth are **non-breastfeeding, post-partum women** with any nutritional risk.

Seventh are individuals at nutritional risk because they are **homeless or migrants**, and **current participants who, without WIC foods, could continue to have medical and/or dietary problems**.

WIC sets stringent criteria for receiving supplemental support, specifically to address the priority nutrition risks. These two major nutritional risk criteria are:
- Medically-based risks such as anemia, underweight, overweight, history of pregnancy complications, or poor pregnancy outcomes.
- Dietary risks, such as failure to meet the dietary guidelines or inappropriate nutrition practices.

Clearly motherhood (not to mention fatherhood) extends far beyond pregnancy, delivery, and care of an infant. While the initial focus for a parent is the physical care of the child, nurses can help focus on nutrition and healthy behaviors from early on by sharing what *services and resources* can help a parent best provide these needs. Helping a mother and father understand available resources in the context of the child and family health should be addressed as early as possible.

Given the economic climate in the U.S. today, nurses must not assume that a family does not need supplemental food assistance. Beyond support from early services like WIC, other federal programs are available for families to assure supplemental food services, but patients may or may not know about them. For example, the USDA Supplemental Nutrition Assistance Program (SNAP) has a set of eligibility criteria and resources to help provide appropriate nutrition for children and families.

According to the USDA, over 21 million households a month (across the nation) participate in the SNAP program (FNS, SNAP, 2012). (This is a dramatic rise from just under 12 million households a month in 2007.) SNAP provides not only monetary support for families, but also funds many of the school programs providing subsidized and free lunches for children. In an attempt to improve the nutrition provided by such programs, the USDA Food and Nutrition Service provides nutritional resources and outreach to the recipients of SNAP and the providers.

Despite the many guides for parents on how to diaper, feed, potty train and socialize a toddler, there are many essential needs of a family that are not highlighted during these early motherhood stages. Parents, often with the highest level of need, can easily fall through the cracks. Nurses can offer information about resources and support, even before they are typically recommended, which can provide an early impetus for healthy choices and needed nutritional aid, be it financial or educational.

References

Amnesty International (2010). Deadly delivery: The maternal health care crisis in the USA March 2010. Retrieved 04/25/12 from https://www.amnesty.org/en/library/info/AMR51/019/2010/en

Ciliberto, C.F., & Marx, G.F., (1998). Physiological Changes Associated with Pregnancy. Update in *Anesthesia Physiology*, Issue 9. Retrieved 12/28/12 from http://www.nda.ox.ac.uk/wfsa/html/u09/u09_003.htm

Mayo Clinic Staff (2012), Heart Conditions and Pregnancy, Know the Risks. Retrieved at Mayo Clinic Website 04/25/12 from http://www.mayoclinic.com/health/pregnancy/PR00124

National Institutes of Health (NIH), (2008). National Institute of Child Health & Human Development. *Gestational Diabetes*. Retrieved 02/29/12 from http://www.nichd.nih.gov/health/topics/gestational_diabetes.cfm

Ruchat, S.M., Davenport, M.H., and Giroux, I. (2012). Nutrition and Exercise Reduce Excessive Weight Gain in Normal-Weight Pregnant Women. *Medicine and Science in Sports & Exercise*. Published ahead of print. doi: 10.1249/MSS.Ob013e31825365f1.

Simmons, D., (2011) Diabetes And Obesity In Pregnancy. *Best Practice & Research Clinical Obstetrics & Gynecology*, Volume 25, Issue 1. Retrieved 11/12 from http://www.bestpracticeobgyn.com/article/S1521-6934(10)00129-X/abstract

United States Department of Agriculture, Food and Nutrition (FNS), (2012) WIC Eligibility Requirements. Retrieved 01/27/12 from http://www.fns.usda.gov/wic/howtoapply/eligibilityrequirements.htm

United States Department of Agriculture, Food and Nutrition (FNS), (2012). Supplemental Nutrition Assistance Program. Retrieved 02/29/12 from http://www.fns.usda.gov/pd/16SNAPpartHH.htm

United States Department of Health and Human Services (HHS), (2012), Maternal Infant and Child Health. Retrieved 04/24/12 from http://www.healthypeople.gov/2020/topicsobjectives2020/overview.aspx?topicid=26

United States Department of Health and Human Services, Health Resources and Service Administration(HHS) (2010). Maternal Morbidity and Risk Factors in Pregnancy. Womens Health USA Retrieved 04/24/12 from http://mchb.hrsa.gov/whusa10/hstat/mh/pages/236mmrfp.html

Chapter 11
Obesity & Older Adults

Over the past few decades, obesity has affected a disproportionate percentage of the older population by age. According to the Center on an Aging Society (2003), in 1991, 75% of the obese population was between ages 51 and 69, while this age group comprised only two-thirds of the population. Although it would seem that the increase in childhood obesity would redistribute the high obesity rates among older adults, the obesity rate among older adults continues to climb (HHS, 2012). Further, it is estimated that by 2030, 60% of the population aged 65 and older will need to manage at least one chronic condition. (*Debbie's note*: from my clinical experience, many older adults with one chronic condition are ultimately diagnosed with more conditions and further complications thereof.) As older adults are the fastest growing segment of the population, with the Baby Boomers first reaching the age of 65 in 2011, illness prevention issues will need to be more thoroughly addressed.

Federal programming, such as Healthy People 2020, recognizes that individual health determinants of older adults, including participation in physical activities and other preventative services, can improve the health outcome of this growing demographic (healthypeople.gov/2020). Preventive services are highly needed, yet are under used by many older adults, especially among certain ethnic and racial populations. Medicare and Medicaid certainly provide highly valuable services, especially among older adults with diabetes in need of chronic medications, glucose-monitoring devices, and assistive devices. Whether you provide the older adult or their caretaker with valuable resources and tools, understanding the health system and resources is paramount to improve the health and quality of life of the aging patient.

> Chapter 11 Objectives:
> 1. Identify trends of obesity among older adults
> 2. Explain the need for and access of preventative care
> 3. Examine common health ailments among older adults
> 4. Recognize how chronic illnesses including depression can affect nutrition and mobility

Based on extensive research and evidence-based practice, the Center for Medicare and Medicaid Services (CMS) decided in 2011 that there was adequate evidence to demonstrate the need for intensive behavioral therapy to prevent and reduce obesity. Now, older adults are entitled to one-on-one face time with a physician or nurse practitioner to screen (using BMI), assess and provide behavioral counseling for obesity and health-related behaviors (CMS, 2011). And it was found that more sessions have been more effective. This change is very significant for the needs of this older population. Realizing that it is not too late to improve health through nutrition, fitness, and modest weight loss or maintenance is a great step in the right direction to improve access to preventative services for older adults.

With these new guidelines, we will likely see a trend towards increased focus on the wellbeing of older adults with obesity and chronic illness. A study by McTigue et. al (2003) conducted a review of literature to answer a few questions regarding the association between obesity, older adults, and morbidity. They found that, yes, obese older adults are at higher risk for certain cardiovascular events, and obesity detection and intervention can be beneficial. The combination of diet, physical activity, and behavioral therapy can improve health. Even modest weight loss can improve health, though the individual's health and nutritional status must be considered, as malnutrition can be easily overlooked in this population. And, of course, physical activity should be modified to fit the unique needs of the patient, depending on underlying chronic illness. Safety and bone health must be considered in the face of activity and weight loss programming for older adults.

As a nurse, whether or not you are specifically familiar with Medicare or Medicaid, you can help direct patients to find services for them. Encouraging older adults to know that they are not forgotten, and are encouraging them to improve their health even in later life, can be helpful. Below is a simplified guide to understanding some differences between Medicare and Medicaid:

Preventative Care: Medicaid vs. Medicare

What is the difference between the two and how can they help my patient?

Table 11-1. Preventative Care: Medicaid vs. Medicare

MEDICARE	MEDICAID
www.medicare.gov 1-800-MEDICARE (633-4227) 1-877-486-2048 (TDD) MyMedicare.gov can help you track covered preventative services & when you received them	www.medicaid.gov Each state has an individual program. A simplified list of 50 US States and Medicaid State Programs can be found at http://www.colorado2.com/medicaid/states.html
>65 years and those with End Stage Kidney Failure	Poor, pregnant women, children, and chronically disabled
Funded by federal government	Joint Funded by Federal and State governments
Medications not generally covered	Medications can be covered
In-hospital care	Long-term and in-home care
Medicare Part A – for hospital bills	Medicaid may pay, but primary insurance pays first
Medicare Part B – for medical insurance	If you have Medicaid and Medicare, Medicaid can help pay your Medicare Part B premium
Medicare Part C – or MA – plan that includes Part A, Part B, part D and may also include vision, dental and hearing. Part C is provided by a private company approved by Medicare	Only some states include dental services in medical. These ancillary services (dental /vision) are the first to be reduced, but are critical for overall health).
Medicare Part D – for prescriptions	Medicaid covers most prescription drugs, and many OTC (over-the-counter). Some cover formulary drugs with certain restrictions
Medigap – supplemental health insurance	Medicaid is a supplemental insurance, but ask about individual need for added supplemental insurance
Obesity Screening & Counseling For BMI>30, may receive obesity counseling in primary care setting	A report from 2008 found that all 50 states provided at least one treatment modality for obesity (nutritional counseling, drug therapy, or bariatric surgery), and 8 states provided all three. Only 10 states were found to provide nutritional and behavioral therapy for children with obesity (Sebelius, 2010).[1]

© 2012 HERO Inc.

II: Obesity & Older Adults

Older adults are at higher risk of chronic conditions, and the impairments and disability that ensue are tremendous. These chronic conditions include arthritis, diabetes, heart disease and dementia. Coronary Artery Disease alone remains a leading cause of death in 84% of adults aged 65 and older (healthypeople.gov, 2012). And, in light of the high incidence of obesity among older adults, and its association with heart disease, the ability of obese older adults to manage multiple and potentially fatal chronic illnesses will further be impaired. The following items show how obesity affects the older adult and obese population:

- **Disability rates are higher among obese older adults**
  Older obese adults are twice as likely to need assistance with multiple activities of daily living (ADLs) than their non-obese counterparts.
  One in three older adults will fall each year, and these falls are the number one cause of preventable death in older adults (healthypeoplc.gov/2020). Falls also lead to increased disability **and inability to remain active and mobile.**
- **Symptoms of chronic illnesses are more severe**
  An obese older patient with arthritis may be *relatively more* debilitated than a non-obese older adult with arthritis.
- **Obese older adults are less likely to exercise that their non-obese cohorts**
  Less than 20% of older adults engage in adequate activity and strength training (www.cdc.gov, 2008). Immobility and lack of access to programs are contributing factors.
- **Obese older adults are less likely to receive help from a caregiver**
  There remains a stigma related to obesity, even among healthcare providers. Unrelated to obesity-related stigma, 1 to 2 million cases of family or caregiver abuse or injury continue.
- **Depression rates are higher as compared to older adults without obesity**
- **A smaller proportion of older adults are still in the workforce**
- **Healthcare expenses are higher among obese older adults**

Complexity of Care

As adults age, their health concerns, risk factors, medication side effects, disabilities, and needs all increase. The complexity regarding their care is due to an intricate web of providers, caregivers, insurance companies, support networks (if they have any), and medications of many kinds. *Polypharmacy* can be an iconic issue for older adults, with upwards of 12 (or more) medications to juggle per day. With nurses to administer medication in a long-term care facility, there is some oversight and monitoring. But for older adults independently juggling a plethora of pills, creams, drops, and ointments, confusion can overwhelm them and lead to noncompliance. With limited mobility, depression, and obesity, a person's ability to care for himself can be diminished even further, leading to a vicious cycle that weakens his health even more.

There is a tendency in medical care to believe that older adults are "too old" for many things, be it chemotherapy for their tumor or fitness for their strength and balance. Every person, old or young, should be assessed on an individual basis, and educated based on his or her needs and ability.

Nurses must understand how obesity complicates the already-complicated chronic illnesses that afflict older adults. But this can potentially be reversed if older adults are willing to maintain, monitor, and/or attempt to control their weight. This is why nurses would be remiss if they fail to encourage patients to adopt healthier patterns even at an old age.

Below is a flowchart to help visualize how obesity can so significantly increase risk and lead to illness, disability and, eventually, premature death.

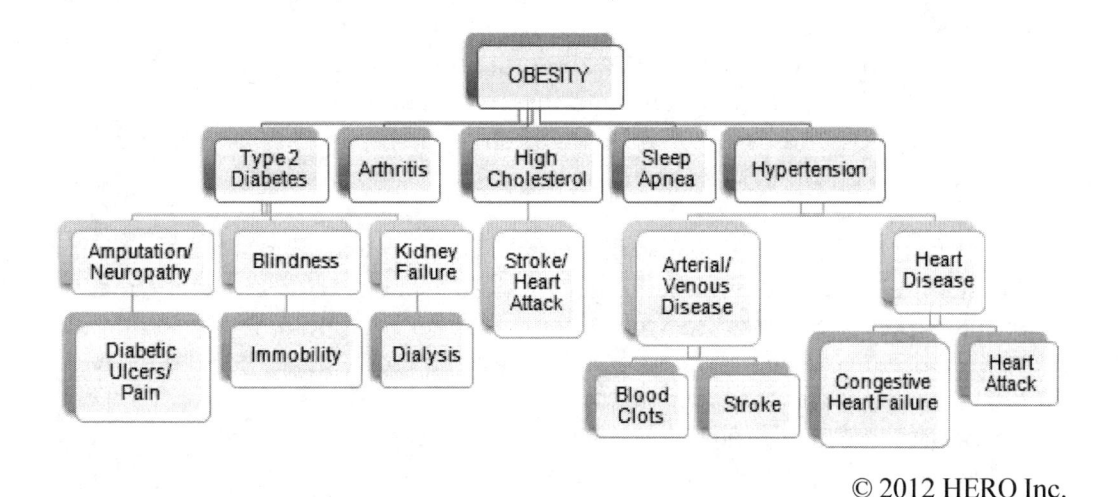

© 2012 HERO Inc.

Figure 11-1. Common Risks of Obesity in the Older Adult

11: Obesity & Older Adults

Common Risks of Obesity in the Older Adult

Unfortunately, heart disease, diabetes, osteoarthritis, hypertension, and high cholesterol are already widespread among older adults. But we must understand two things:

1. Obesity increases the likelihood of each of these conditions, and
2. All of these conditions are not normal to aging, though they are common

Obesity and the Care of the Older Adult: *Mobility*

Again, it would be easy for nurses and caretakers to assume that older adults are too old and frail for physical activity, and too set in their ways to adopt healthier food choices and palates. But this would be shortsighted. While mobility is *already* impaired among older adults, obesity worsens the individual's mobility even further, which is why exercise may help. Nurses should help the older adult and family understand the need for continued mobility and exercise by asking the following questions:

- What was their prior level of activity? What type of activity interests them?
- What are the limitations? Do they rely on a walker, wheelchair, etc.?
- What are reasonable activity goals for the patient?
    - Can the older adult walk to the restroom and back?
    - Possible goal: 3 trips to the kitchen and back a day
- What type of care is available for the patient? Family, caregiver?
- Compliance: is the patient willing to carryout exercises?

Understanding the older adult's living situation, whether at home or in a nursing facility, is essential to helping set mobility goals. Unfortunately, many older adults lack the needed services to enable them to remain active. Without needed medical care, nursing support, and family support, many older adults end up disabled, bedridden, and dependent.

Nurses must understand how the nursing care of older adults will be impacted by obesity. Obesity of the older adult will not only impair the patient, but the caregiver or nurse as well. The following chart gives some relevant examples.

Table 11-2. Impact of Obesity on Nursing Care of the Older Hospitalized Patient

Nursing Task	Impact of Obesity
Imaging X Rays, CT scan, MRI	Limited ability to penetrate subcutaneous fat, size constraints of closed MRI, scanners
Medication IM injections oral doses wound care barrier creams	Typical IM needle may not reach muscle through thick subcutaneous fat, reduced efficacy of medication doses, increased surface area for topical creams, slowed healing, more barrier cream due to friction
Mobility by Patient Walkers, wheelchair, motorized wheelchair	Greater need for assisted mobility devices due to arthritis, diabetes, breathing trouble, heart disease and obesity
Caretaker and Mobility: ability to lift and maneuver patient	Physically challenging to care for an obese older adult with ADL needs, toileting, bedpan
Increased Complexity of Chronic Illness	Managing chronic conditions exacerbated by obesity: diabetes, heart disease, depression
Size of Gowns and Equipment	Require larger BP cuffs, beds, chairs, commodes, clothing
Nutrition Services	Require more nutritional consultation
Physical Therapy	Require greater physical therapy and rehabilitative support

© 2012 HERO Inc.

Nutrition and the Older Adult

Nutrition is a significant challenge for many older adults regardless of weight. As many older adults carry diagnoses of diabetes, heart disease, and dementia, multiple issues complicate the nutritional intake of the individual. The acute medical condition, or even the chronic condition, often overwhelms the patient and caretaker enough that nutrition gets little direct attention.

Even though we, as nurses, understand that metabolism slows as we age, and we therefore require fewer calories, many of our patients do not understand this and will continue to eat as they did in their earlier years. Or, medical conditions might affect their nutrition in so many ways that they are at a loss as to what to eat, when and why. Consider an obese man with diabetes and heart disease, now treated for congestive heart failure. Between a low sugar diet for diabetes, low fat and low sodium diet for the heart, and now also a water restricted diet for the heart failure, unless the patient is cared for by a medical dietitian inhouse, what is he to eat? He already likely is not so mobile, lives in a "food desert" with few shops nearby, and can only buy processed food… now what?

Making the best possible choices at any given time requires the knowledge to do so. Choosing nutrient-dense foods can help provide more nutrition with fewer calories in order to maximize nutrition. Also, as digestive processes slow, eating foods high in fiber becomes more important. Finally, a wide variety of foods should continue to be eaten, as this is the best way to ingest the required vitamins and minerals, which are essential for many conditions including wound healing, improving the senses of taste and smell, and bone health. See the following table for more information.

Table 11-3. Nutrition For Older Adults

WHAT	WHY
PLENTY OF WATER	Thirst diminishes, but the need for water remains high. Helps prevent constipation
LEAN MEATS and FISH	Many older adults already have high cholesterol. Muscle mass is lost in older age.
LOW SODIUM and SALT	To help control high blood pressure and heart disease
HIGH VITAMINS and ELECTROLYTES	Many heart medications alter the natural balance
HIGH FIBER	Digestion slows, leaving one prone to constipation
VARIETY OF FRUITS and VEGETABLES	Increases fiber, vitamins, water
VARIETY OF TEXTURES	To increase appearance of food if appetite is low. Dentition may limit ability to chew. Swallow ability may diminish with dementia or stroke. Blended or minced food may be needed
INCREASE CALCIUM and VITAMIN D	Low bone density and little access to sunlight. Drinking low fat milk is good

© 2012 HERO Inc

Sometimes a patient, either following a stroke or with severe dementia, may not be able to tolerate thin liquids like water or juice. Altering the consistency is crucial for safety and to prevent aspiration into the lungs, a potentially life-threatening complication.

Depending on the needs and frailty of the older adult, referral to a speech pathologist may be necessary for swallow evaluation. Powdered thickeners can help modify foods to make them easier to swallow. Having older adults sit up properly to eat, and providing the proper texture of food are both crucial elements among frail older adults.

In addition to specific needs for mechanically providing appropriate nutrition, access to foods becomes more difficult as people age. Consider the following reasons:

- Is the older adult able to drive?
- Are there stores nearby?
- Does the person need help to shop? If so, does he have help to shop?
- Does the patient have proper dentition? Are teeth in good repair? Or does he have suitable dentures?
- Is the patient cognitively capable of keeping food safe and fresh in the home?
- What social services are available to the older adult? Meals on Wheels? Shopping assistance?
- Is the patient on a salt restricted diet? If so, what about compliance?
- Is the patient on a diabetic diet? If so, is he compliant?
- How often does he test his blood sugar? Does a nurse visit?
- Does the patient have someone to share meals with? Or does he eat alone?
- Does he have dementia? Does he remember to eat?

How Depression Affects the Older Adult and Wellness

Depression is the most under-recognized, under-diagnosed, and under-treated condition among older adults, with a disproportionately high percentage of American older adults dying due to depression-related suicide. In 2004, 14.3 out of 100,000 people age 65 and over died by suicide. This is higher than the suicide rate of the general population, which is 11 people per 100,000. We know that depression is higher among people with chronic illnesses, and 80% of adults over age 65 have at least one chronic condition (CDC, 2012), so perhaps it is no surprise that these two conditions have converged in such a way.

Because of the complexity of dealing with adults with numerous illnesses and numerous medications, depression may be confused with medication side effects or other conditions. In addition, depression is sometimes mistaken for dementia, but if it were correctly diagnosed as depression, it could be more easily treated. However, if left untreated, depression can lead to lack of appetite, lack of interests, antisocial behavior, lethargy and, of course, suicide.

Though depression and depressive symptoms are *not* a normal part of aging, feelings of grief from losing friends and any disability from an underlying chronic illness can contribute to depression. Depending on the health of the patient, his ability to remain active in the workforce, his ability to remain social, and his support network, an older adult may struggle with feelings of helplessness and an overall lack of self worth. The Geriatric Depression Scale is an easy tool to administer as an initial assessment of depression. One of the YES/NO questions asks whether the older adult has dropped many of their usual activities or interests (Sheikh et al, 1991).

If the lack of activity is due to depression rather than mobility or access, then intervention should be provided to help the older adult regain the mental desire to become active again. While depression is not specifically related to obesity, nutrition or fitness, depression will certainly impede healthful behaviors in an older adult.

Despite certain significant considerations for nutrition and activity for older adults, many older adults remain quite active and healthful into their older years. Explaining how they are successfully maintaining their health through adequate fitness and nutrition can help further their well being. Therefore, it's imperative that we encourage older adults to continue to make smart food choices and to be as active and mobile as possible.

Summary

While the limitations of many older adults must be considered, the older population requires the same healthy behaviors as their younger counterparts. Nurses must encourage healthy eating, physical activity, and healthy behaviors for adults aged 65 and older, regardless of underlying chronic illness and debility. A variety of reasons might dissuade nurses from actively promoting health, especially in the face of existing immobility, frailty, obesity, and/or heart and lung disease. Nurses are encouraged to tell older patients that even nominal healthy behaviors can improve their well being. Knowing that the risk of falls is outweighed by the benefit of mobility should encourage nurses to take active (and safe) measures to implement activity for their older patients. While more support might be needed, physically and socially, to implement healthy changes, nurses should lead the way to health through referral and encouragement to access health resources.

References

Centers for Disease Control (CDC), 2012, Depression is not a Normal Part of Growing Older. Retrieved 06/07/12 at http://www.cdc.gov/aging/mentalhealth/depression.htm

Centers for Medicare and Medicare Services (CMS), (2011). Decision Memo for Intensive Behavioral Therapy for Obesity. Retrieved 05/07/12 from http://www.cms.gov/medicare-coverage-database/details/nca-decision-memo.aspx?&NcaName=Intensive%20Behavioral%20Therapy%20for%20Obesity&bc=ACAAAAAIAAA&NCAId=253&

McTigue, K., Harris, R., Hemphill, M.B., Bunton, A.J., Lux, L.J., Sutton, S. and Lohr, K.N. (2003) Screening and Interventions for Obesity in Adults: Summary of the Evidence for the U.S. Preventive Services Task Force. *Annals of Internal Medicine*. pp 933-949.

Ruchat ,S.M., Davenport, M.H., Giroux, I., Hillier, M., Batada, A., Sopper, M.M., Hammond, J.A., Mottola, M.F. (2012). Nutrition and Exercise Reduce Excessive Weight Gain in Normal-Weight Pregnant Women. *Australian Journal of Science and Medicine in Sport*. March 26, 2012 [Epub ahead of print].

Sebelius, K. (2010). Secretary of Health and Human Services. Preventive and Obesity-Related Services Available to Medicaid Enrollees. Retrieved 05/08/12 from http://www.medicaid.gov/Medicaid-CHIP-Program-Information/By-Topics/Quality-of-Care/Downloads/RTC_PreventiveandObesityRelatedServices.pdf

Sheikh, J.I., Yesavage, J.A., Brooks, III, J.O., Friedman, L.F., Gratzinger, P., Hill, R.D., Zadeik, A. and Crook, T. (1991): Proposed factor structure of the Geriatric Depression Scale. *International Psychogeriatrics*. 3: 23-28.

United States Department of Health and Human Services (HHS), (2012), Older Adults. Retrieved 01/24/12 from http://www.healthypeople.gov/2020/topicsobjectives2020/overview.aspx?topicid=26

PART IV: PLAN

      Thus far, this Guide has walked us through the Subjective, Objective and Assessment portions of our nursing care plan related to obesity. After the completion of the patient assessment, it is time to develop a comprehensive plan and strategy to address the causative factors of obesity. The culmination of a lack of nutrition and physical activity must be addressed and reversed. We learned how to identify a patient as a unique individual with intrinsic and extrinsic influences. We learned how to monitor, measure, and physically examine the patient to learn how signs, symptoms and underlying illnesses or disability can affect obesity and weight. Furthermore, we learned how to assess the situation to determine the degree of obesity, and its relationship to the patient's overall health condition in all its forms. Now, we must create a realistic plan. Once the patient steps beyond our office, hospital setting, or outpatient clinic, we must acknowledge that they may not return for follow-up.

      A nursing plan must be well designed to foster compliance and to empower the patient to continue along a path to improvement.

Part IV Objectives:

1. Learn how to set realistic nutritional and dietary goals
2. Understand how to plan slow and steady fitness goals
3. Learn how to empower each patient to "Be Your Own HERO©"

Chapter 12
Nutrition & Obesity in Daily Life

While the aim of The HERO Guide To Health is obesity prevention through health promotion and *not weight loss*, per se, we must discuss various ways of helping those who are already overweight or obese. We must clarify that "thin" does not mean "healthy," and likewise "obese" is not synonymous with "unhealthy" (though we aim to educate on the health risks associated with obesity). Perhaps this is why many overweight adults may struggle with initiating healthier habits. If an overweight or obese person without illness appears and feels "healthy," they may not have the drive or feel the need to change habits. Conversely, they might feel that their ability to change is a "lost cause."

As nurses, we must recognize all the factors that contribute to the rise in obesity among any and all populations. We learned already how to assess the unique individual, but we must also understand how the interventions and plans are similarly affected by socioeconomic issues like education, race, and socioeconomic status. Unfortunately, whether or not a patient will receive counseling or even acknowledge their obesity has been determined already, in part, by their socioeconomic status and ethnicity. Ironically, the health disparity in terms of prevalence of obesity according to race is declining, though the actual disparity of receiving care remains.

> Chapter 12 Objectives:
> 1. Support that ALL individuals should focus on health promotion
> 2. Plan how to make simple and effective changes even with limited resources
> 3. Describe a few popular diets and assess their differences

A study by Zhang and Wang (2004) used data from National Health and Nutrition Examination Surveys (NHANES) to analyze over 28,000 people (ages 20 to 60) between 1971 and 2000, and showed the equalizing of obesity prevalence across race. While the relative difference in disparity among three socioeconomic groups (low, medium, and high) was 50% in 1971, it had decreased to a relative disparity of 14% by 2000. Study findings conclude that socio-environmental influences appear greater than the influence of individual characteristics of the person. This means that, although lower socioeconomic status often increases risk of disease processes for a variety of reasons, no cohort is immune to obesity, even among higher socioeconomic groups. This emphasizes the need to provide education and intervention across ALL socioeconomic groups. But how can we equalize the access and use of interventions for certain populations who may otherwise not receive necessary obesity prevention?

This is why our HERO program, though focusing initially on lower socioeconomic groups, provides outreach to the communities at large. HERO recognizes that obesity does not occur in a vacuum, nor can anyone become immune to it. Intervention must be offered to all, though greater intervention is required for those with greater contributing factors.

According to the Agency for Healthcare and Research and Quality Survey (2002-2007), despite slight improvement from 2002 to 2007 regarding percentages of people who receive counseling on healthy eating (48.9% to 51.6% respectively), disparities among populations who receive the counseling remain. Adults age 18-44 were least likely to receive advice about healthy eating. And poorer individuals, those with less than a high school education, or Hispanics compared to Whites, were less likely to receive counseling on healthy eating and exercise. Strikingly, in 2007, for obese adults, 52.7% of poor compared to 66.6% of high income adults received counseling on the need for exercise. Survey data from 2005-2008 showed that 65.9% of obese adults aged 20 and over reported being told by a doctor or health professional that they were overweight or obese (AHRQ, 2012).

The percentage of overweight people who are told they are overweight appears to increase by age. This means that a doctor is more likely to tell a parent of an 8-year-old that the child is overweight than the doctor is to tell the parent that a 3-year-old the same thing.

- Are clinicians shirking the subject among younger patients, hoping that growth curves will stabilize?
- Are clinicians now understanding more about the health consequences of early intervention for obesity?
- Policies to monitor younger and counsel younger patients will surely be needed to equalize education and intervention for all groups of all ages.

(AHRQ, 2012)

We must understand that ALL of us should strive for healthier nutrition and fitness habits. Overweight and obese adults *still* have the ability for obesity prevention measures, though the process is likely more challenging and lengthy. Consistent medical evidence shows that obesity increases the risk of many cancers, increases the recurrence rate, and decreases the overall survival from cancer. Therefore, especially among people who are already obese, the need for improved health and body weight should be seen still as prevention and health promotion (Rock, et al 2012).

Understanding WHY fitness and nutrition is needed *even* and *especially* if one is already overweight or obese is essential. And HOW to do this successfully is the greatest challenge. Many people have been known to successfully lose weight then "yo-yo" back, and are unable to maintain the new improved weight they tried so hard to attain. Why does this happen? Perhaps, if changes are too drastic and weight loss is too fast, the plan is not realistic for that person. Setting realistic goals that are sustainable and have appropriate expectations for that person will lead to the best success. And remember that success does not necessarily mean losing a specific amount of weight or reaching a certain BMI. Weight loss success should be measured according to the person's ability to make lasting dietary changes, even if less weight was lost than desired.

We can safely say that weight loss and changing dietary patterns is not an easy task. Naturally, people want to see immediate results, or are challenged by the changes that should be continued long-term, and thus give up prematurely. Whether you read this as a nurse, parent, friend, or co-worker, you have taken the first, hardest step towards helping yourself or others. Honesty, patience, knowledge, and self-determination are the critical elements of any successful plan. HERO does not claim to be a weight loss program, but rather we use basic health knowledge to provide straightforward and common sense solutions to combat obesity on a daily basis. We will also discuss the pros and cons of various commercially-available diet plans, and will show a "sample" seven-day nutrition plan (written by HERO program co-founder, Debbie Kantor) to encourage and to simplify the daunting prospect of changing one's eating habits. Weight loss should be realistic and not drastic, inclusive and not restrictive, and long term not short term. We prefer not the term "diet" but rather a "health pattern." Unfortunately, the term "diet" tends to connote a quick crash diet that is both severely restrictive and not often sustainable. To best implement an effective health pattern, nutritional and fitness changes must be implemented *over time*. Behaviors must be relatively consistent and changes must also be *maintained*. And continued education regarding the health benefits of improved nutrition and fitness can help encourage the continued health pattern.

While "slow and steady" can win the race to health, the lengthy process of weight loss without seeing significant or rapid responses can be frustrating and discouraging. Because of America's culture of treatment and "quick fix" solutions, a discouraged person might resort to fad diets, weight loss pills or supplements, or even more severe treatment like bariatric surgery. Without knowing the health risks or actual need for these treatments, results can be even less effective, and sometimes even more detrimental to one's health. Remember the issues with weight loss pills in the 1990s? Over a decade and many class-action lawsuits later, many of these pills were reportedly responsible for heart attacks, heart conditions, and even death. For the first time in years, a new weight loss medication is nearing approval by the Food and Drug Administration, and time will tell the efficacy and safety of this medication. But just as we recommend getting vitamins and minerals directly from our foods rather than via supplements, it should be recommended by health practitioners to first find a suitable and sustainable health pattern before opting for a quick fix with an unknown results. As a nurse, offering accurate health information, providing needed referrals and resources, and continuing to encourage the patient can improve their drive to remain compliant to succeed with a plan.

Unfortunately, American society and the mainstream media set high, extreme, and often unachievable goals for weight loss and "normal" size. Fad or crash diets advertise extreme weight loss by individuals (who are sometimes only depicted by actors) and set unrealistic and sometimes unhealthy goals. Helping your patient to recognize the unrealistic media presentation of weight loss is necessary for individualized and sustainable long-term weight loss or health improvement.

For instance, emphasizing why losing 60 pounds in the next two months may not be practical, possible, or recommended should be addressed. As a nurse, you can help encourage your patients to find a suitable way to make slow and sustainable changes that fit into their social environment and schedule. The ability to make needed health changes is tremendously difficult at best, and social situations can exacerbate the struggle. This is why nurses can really make a difference and provide another level of both reality and encouragement.

Because fad diets (not to mention many commercially-available diets, which will be discussed later in the chapter) promise great results, it can be difficult to interest patients in the long-term health solutions that truly help. Patients need to be assured that even small steps are improving health even if **weight loss** is not immediately accomplished, as this may give the patient some positives to work with as he or she attempts to lose weight.

What Changes are Needed?

Nurses must help patients understand the goals of changing health patterns. Goals may include a combination of the following:

- **To lose weight and thus lower BMI**
- **To improve overall health**
- **To decrease symptoms such as sleep apnea, joint pain, mobility issues**
- **To prevent/control Type 2 diabetes**
- **To lower blood pressure**
- **Lastly … to set REALISTIC GOALS**

Lean Times and a Call to Action

Another problem with weight management, paradoxically, is the current economy. Because many people today are struggling during difficult financial times, they may not be able to eat well or nutritionally on a consistent basis. Some people, even in their 70s and 80s, must now return to work to pay for their health care expenses. Other, younger, people may return to the workforce when they otherwise may have been able to stay home with their children. Still others are out of work and have needed to "cut back" and change their lifestyles. And finally, for those who still have jobs, many now work *multiple* jobs in order to afford food and expenses for the family. All of this makes eating a far harder challenge than it should be.

Consider this: due to the current economic challenges, a family that otherwise may have sat down for dinner together may now need to go their separate ways at meal times to accommodate altered shift work. This means that some, if not all, of the family will have to take many more meals outside the home than ever before. And some of those may not have the energy to first shop, prepare, then bag lunches for the family members who must work more hours away from home – or be unable to pay their bills.

Whatever the reason for changes in employment and finances, the majority of people in this country are affected in some way or another. When work patterns change, so do eating habits and activity levels, which is why the need to discuss healthy nutritional strategies has become so important.

We know that effective nurses must wear many "hats." We are a caregiver, advisor, confidant, educator, and professional with a broadened human perspective. In what ways can nurses offer sound advice for health promotion, while still remaining sensitive to people's financial struggles?

While it might seem beyond a nurse's scope to offer certain advice related to finances, we offer a few suggestions that relate back to the patient's health and wellbeing:

Sample Scenario

Ms. P. is 46 years old ad works 9 a.m. to 5 p.m. at a desk job for a business office in order to earn a meager salary. She is a single mother with two children, 6 and 9, and knows she is overweight. She is frustrated by trying many "diets" and has essentially given up. Her desire to lose weight eats at her, but she feels she just can't do it.

She returns from work exhausted, rarely has time to shop for fresh foods, and has little money to spend on "health foods." Mostly, she eats out from fast food restaurants while at work, and feeds her children prepared foods at home (frozen pizza is their staple). She wants to eat better, but does not know how and she never exercises and mostly drives from Point A to Point B.

She worries her children will become overweight, too, especially because her 9-year-old daughter is already the largest girl in her class. Ms. P. wants help for the family, but doesn't have a plan.

***

What can we gather from this scenario?
- Ms. P. is struggling financially
- Ms. P. is overworked
- Ms. P. needs more support
- Ms. P. knows she needs help

With this amount of information, the nurse can already help formulate a plan *with*, not *for*, Ms. P. The nurse can see that the main issues are finances, eating patterns, and the lack of exercise.

Ideally, beginning to pack food from home can reduce some calories, sodium, and fat, while also reducing cost. Packing a turkey sandwich on whole grain bread and a banana even *once* a week can be a realistic start to both reduce cost and reduce calories, sodium and fat.

Many people feel that changing eating habits must be "all or nothing," but this is a daunting, tricky, and often short-lived way to make changes. By suggesting even a small change, you can encourage Mrs. P. that even one day a week can make a difference to both cost and improved eating habits.

Even if Ms. P. continues to eat fast-food lunches every day, you can still encourage small changes. Are any of these restaurants within walking distance? Encouraging a **short walk** instead of car ride (weather-permitting) can be a good start toward helping Ms. P. gain some needed fitness and improving her health in the process.

Encouraging Ms. P. to **keep a food journal** of the food she buys for lunch can help make her more aware of the nutritional content of her choices, which may also help.

If Ms. P. is willing to substitute a few foods on the fast-food menu for her current choices, this can help, while not too rapidly, to change her patterns. For example, if she normally orders a **double** cheeseburger, she should substitute a **single** burger instead. If she orders **large** fries, encourage her to order **small** fries instead. If she orders a **sugared soda**, encourage her to order a **smaller size, diet soda or drink water,** as all three options are increasingly better choices.

> **NOTE:** The issue of sugared drinks versus artificial sweeteners is complex, depending on the goal of the dietary changes. If the goal is to reduce calories, removing sugared drinks can help. If the goal is to drink natural, not artificial, beverages, water remains the best option.

Together, you can write a lunch plan for Ms. P., even if fast food is her only option. A **concrete plan** can be easier to follow at first. Discuss what Ms. P. feels she is willing and able to change. Don't expect her to suddenly give up burgers for salad, as that is unrealistic. Baby steps work best.

> **NOTE:** This plan is used to begin making healthier choices. While soda and cheeseburgers are not advocated, the point is that small steps to modify an existing diet may help encourage small changes, which will reduce empty calories and fat and thus improve overall health.

A sample plan may look like this:

Table 12-1. Sample Meal Plan for Beginners

Monday	Tuesday	Wednesday	Thursday	Friday
Small Soda & water	Small Diet Soda & water	Water	Small Diet Soda & water	Water
Grilled Chicken Sandwich	Value Burger (usually $1 or so)	Grilled Chicken Salad	Turkey wrap/sub Choose 6", not 12"	Value cheeseburger
Fruit side	Side salad	Value fries	Fruit side	Side salad

The goals of following such a menu are:
- Drinking more water than before
- Ordering smaller-sized burgers
- Introducing fruit or salad as a side, rather than fries with every sandwich
- Encouraging alternating choices
- Reducing weekly food cost (value burgers are smaller and cost less)
- Asking for a cup of ice water two out of every five work days saves 40% of drink expenses

Involving Ms. P.'s children in some of her food planning can help make health and nutrition a family priority. According to nutrition studies and social learning theory, when children see their parents eating well, they will be more likely to do so, as well (Nnakwe, 2009).

Using the foundations from the USDA's choosemyplate.gov, nurses can refer patients to simple guides without preaching a specific plan.

Dietary Plans: Pros and Cons

That said, some patients might still ask their nurse, "which diet is best?" Of course, depending on the patient's baseline health and medical needs, and ability to follow a certain diet, some patients might ask your opinion of a commonly practiced diet. Below, we discuss a few currentlyavailable commercial diet plans, as it might help to guide your patients toward the best diet plan for them. You can help them understand the basic framework of these diets. For the most part, increasing vegetables, whole grains, lean protein, and fiber, while decreasing fats and sugars are common among them.

Twenty-five popular diets were rated by *US News and World Report* (Comarow, 2012) and were ranked by twenty-two experts in the field of diet, nutrition, and exercise.

The best overall diet, and the one that was ranked the best for healthy eating, is the DASH diet. Designed by the National Heart, Lung, and Blood Institute (NHLBI), the DASH diet, Dietary Approaches to Stop Hypertension, was designed to lower cholesterol and high blood pressure. But encouraging whole grains, fruits, vegetables, fiber, and protein also helps reduce the waistline. Since it was designed by a federal program, the plan is available for free online, which may prove helpful to economically-stressed patients.

The US News and World Report ranked the best diet for weight loss, the easiest diet plan to follow, and the best commercially-available plan as the Weight Watchers® plan.

Weight Watchers® uses a point system to help people focus on the number of calories consumed to help lose weight. Depending on age, weight, and gender, people use the point system (PointsPlus®) to track points throughout the day. Foods like fresh fruits and vegetables have no points and, thus, can be eaten freely, while foods with empty calories have high points assigned.

In the Weight Watchers® plan, nutritionally dense foods are encouraged over others, though any foods can be eaten when sticking within a target's total points. A database containing 40,000 points enables people to easily research point values for any foods they eat. This program essentially is a calorie-counting program, but with an easily followed format and a support system to encourage people along.

The main drawback to the Weight Watchers® plan in these tough economic times is the expense. There is a fee for meetings and *e-tool* access, though attending meetings can improve compliance.

The number one ranked diabetic diet was the Biggest Loser diet. With the popularity of the reality television series of the same name, and the ability to watch people successfully see results, the Biggest Loser diet has gained momentum and popularity. Focusing on the two essentials, calorie restriction and fitness, this diet is likely to lead to weight loss.

In the case of all of these diets, the ease with which media can help to spread success stories likely contributes to the more popular diet programs. Following what is known of Social Learning Theory, people are more likely to make health improvements when they observe a group around them attempting the same. Programs that help boost morale by showing real people with very real stories, and their battles with obesity, can lead to a greater impact on society and obesity. These examples of mainstream diet programs are included in order to have a basic idea of programs your patients may ask you about.

The context of the person's condition and the primary goal must be incorporated into his or her plan. The nurse also must emphasize, again, that there is **no quick fix**. While improving eating and fitness programs are certainly valuable, there remain health risks related to genetics, our environment, and uncertainties in life, which is why emphasizing long-term solutions is essential.

References

Comarow, A. (2012). Best Diets Methodology: How we rated 25 eating plans. *US News and World Report*. E-publication, January, 3. Retrieved 02/28/12 from http://health.usnews.com/best-diet/articles/2012/01/03/best-diets-methodology-how-we-rated-25-eating-plans

Nnakwe, N (2008). *Community nutrition: planning health promotion and disease prevention*. Jones and Bartlett Publishers, MA, USA.

Rock, C. L., Doyle, C., Demark-Wahnefried, W., Meyerhardt, J., Courneya, K. S., Schwartz, A. L., Bandera, E. V., Hamilton, K. K., Grant, B., McCullough, M., Byers, T. and Gansler, T. (2012), Nutrition and physical activity guidelines for cancer survivors. *A Cancer Journal for Clinicians*. doi: 10.3322/caac.21142. Retrieved 04/26/12 from http://onlinelibrary.wiley.com/doi/10.3322/caac.21142/full

United States Department of Health and Human Services (HHS) and Agency for Healthcare Research and Quality (AHRQ) (2009). National Healthcare Disparities Report. Retrieved 04/10/12 from http://www.ahrq.gov/qual/nhdr10/Chap2c.htm#lifestyle

United States Department of Health and Human Services (HHS) and Agency for Healthcare Research and Quality (AHRQ) (2009). National Healthcare Disparities Report. Retrieved 01/16/12 from http://www.ahrq.gov/qual/qrdr09/6_maternalchildhealth/T6_4_4-1.htm

Zhang, Q, and Wang, Y. (2004). Trends in the association between obesity and socioeconomic status in U.S. adults: 1971 to 2000. *Obesity Research Journal*. Retrieved 03/12/12 from http://www.ncbi.nlm.nih.gov/pubmed/15536226

Chapter 13
Fitness Plans: When, How & Why

"Physical fitness is not only one of the most important keys to a healthy body, it is the basis of dynamic and creative intellectual activity."
— John F. Kennedy

In the context of fitness and physical activity, it is imperative to bring together all facets of the previous chapters: understanding the problem, diagnosing the condition and assessing the individual needs of the patient, in order to proceed to the next stage of developing a plan of action. The information collated from previous chapters will provide a baseline for a personal strategic plan, which will include,

- Where the patient has come from,
- Where they are now and
- What they want to achieve.

This chapter will help create clear, concise goals that are both realistic, achievable and important in a health development plan. These goals should be incremental, with each new goal achievement laying the foundation for the next. In this chapter, we specifically look at fitness and physical activities and strategies for incorporating exercise into personal routines by addressing:

- Frequency of exercise,
- Where to exercise and
- Types of exercise.

Physical fitness is important at any age, and contributes not only to the development and maintenance of a healthy weight, but also decreases the likelihood of obesity-related illnesses (including high cholesterol, diabetes, and heart disease) (CDC, 2006). In this chapter, we will discuss the various beneficial aspects of fitness, and why it's imperative to engage in some type of physical activity throughout all stages of life.

> **NOTE:** The word "fitness" means a great many different things to a great many people. For the purposes of this chapter, consider its primary meaning to be one of "beneficial, healthy exercise."

13: Fitness Plans: When, How & Why

> **Chapter 13 Objectives:**
> 1. Outline recommendations for fitness at different ages
> 2. Explain how to safely exercise and build fitness gradually
> 3. Discuss the difference between moderate and vigorous exercise

While healthcare professionals already know that exercise improves muscle tone and cardiovascular endurance, it may also have the capacity to improve mental alertness, as well as fight depression and improve self-esteem. (Otto, M., and Smits, J. 2011)

In the preliminary stages of a health examination, it is imperative to determine what the patient actually believes "healthy exercise" is – you might be surprised by the answers, and this is why a patient's attitude toward exercise is extremely important. For many patients, you will see that the word "fitness" comes with many negative connotations that may include pain, past poor performance, or even the mistaken belief often summed up as "no pain, no gain." A significant proportion of the patients you will assess have not been physically active for some time, because of these very same negative connotations.

Attitudes toward fitness have been formed over many years. People often think about prior experiences, whether it is high school gym class where they might have been forced to climb a perilously high rope while being screamed at by a coach, compulsory track where they couldn't stop unless it was to be sick, or a sport that brings back memories of painful injuries. All of these various past experiences may be part of why the patient either doesn't exercise enough, or doesn't exercise at all.

No matter what connotation is associated with the word "fitness," health professionals should emphasize the benefits of regular physical activity to whatever ability their patients can achieve. Fitness and exercise play a crucial part in battling obesity and its co-morbidities (Poirier, et al 2001). Remember again that the goal of fitness must be understood. If the goal is weight loss, the fitness routine will vary from a routine with the goal of muscle building, toning, improving flexibility, or preventing heart disease. Though, often, increasing fitness can accomplish multiple goals at the same time. Healthy eating and active living are synonymous with, and must be used in conjunction with, one another in order to reverse the effects of obesity.

Fitness is important, yes, but it must be supplemented with dietary changes (as indicated previously) in order to reverse the effects of obesity.

The challenge for many is how to modify an already set schedule and health habits. The path of "least resistance," if they are already not physically active, takes less energy than introducing new behaviors that require new schedules and activities. Sometimes, basic health education to understand why fitness and nutritional changes are needed must be accomplished before there is enough understanding, or inspiration, to adhere to these beneficial new behaviors.

Regardless of your personal opinion towards exercise, encouraging people to be active in any capacity is vital. As a nursing professional you are encouraged to *educate*, *facilitate*, and help patients establish healthy goals that are both realistic and achievable. Note that you are *not* expected to perform the duties of a personal trainer for each patient, nor in each case are you expected to show each patient a range of exercises or to write up a prolonged fitness plan; that is simply unrealistic and not truly within a nurse's scope.

Nurses can help patients to understand *how* and *why* regular physical activity can improve their health and quality of life. This includes those who have chronic illnesses and/or disabilities; as we said in Chapter 7; it's *more* important for a disabled person, or someone dealing with chronic health problems, to get whatever exercise he or she can tolerate than it is for another person to do so.

According to Healthy People 2020, adults and older adults should exercise to reduce the risk of the following:

- Early death
- Coronary artery disease
- Stroke
- Diabetes
- Depression
- Osteoporosis

For children and adolescents, physical fitness can:
- Improve bone health
- Improve cardio, respiratory, and muscle health
- Reduce body fat
- Reduce depression

(HealthyPeople.gov, 2012)

Although the frequency of recommended physical activity varies according to the source, most federal guidelines (like the USDA, CDC, and Department of Health and Human Services) agree that children and adults should strive for exercise most days of the week. But this exercise, especially for the disabled and for older adults, should be to tolerance – not to the point of muscle failure, as this only discourages people who may have just started to exercise after a long period of inactivity.

The U.S. Department of Health and Human Services guidelines list the following regarding how frequently someone should exercise for maximum health benefits:

- **Children** aged 6-17 should be physically active **60 minutes a day**, with most of the 60 minutes involving moderate to vigorous exercise.
- Non-disabled adults aged 18-64 should maintain 2 hours and 30 minutes of exercise a week, with two of the days incorporating moderate or vigorous exercise. (They further point out that, if you increase your activity level to 5 hours of fitness a week, there are additional health benefits.)
- Older adults should follow the adult guidelines to the best of their abilities.
- Children and adults with disabilities should consult with their providers to follow the most suitable and beneficial fitness plan that won't exacerbate their underlying health issues.

(Adapted from Health.gov, 2012)

How Much Exercise, and How Often?

Recommending an hour of physical activity per day may seem somewhat excessive for many of your patients, but by an hour a day, we don't mean that it has to happen all at once. Exercise can be conducted in increments (we are not expecting people to magically start running an hour a day), as this might be much easier for a previously inactive person to tolerate. This exercise can be walking, taking stairs, housecleaning, dancing, or any other activity that increases the heart rate.

Doing small activities 6 times per day for 10 minutes is not unrealistic for most people. (Patients who deal with physical disabilities which involve mobility issues may wish to try "chair exercises," such as "marching in place" while they sit, and various arm and trunk movements.) Any exercise, though, is good exercise; dependent upon the physical capacity of your patient, 30 minutes a day may be a significant increase in his or her daily activity level. *More is not always better.* Consistency and safety are more important, so be sure that starting out working *too* hard does not lead to injury that will disrupt the patient's ability to exercise consistently.

In the fitness world, there is a plethora of conflicting literature that confuses people not only regarding exercise itself, but also on what to eat, when to eat and how to eat it. When dealing with consumption-based weight loss diets, people can find calorie-based systems, low carbohydrate diets, multicultural diets from around the world, and a multitude of restrictive diets ranging from soup to red meat. This is confusing and adds an additional level of complexity that patients just starting an exercise program do not need. While other chapters of <u>The HERO Guide to Health</u> go into significant nutrition detail, as a healthcare professional, it is important that you express basic concepts as simply as possible and not allow the patient to delve quickly into a quick fix mentality.

It is important for the patient to understand that exercise burns calories and that, to lose weight, you must burn calories. And exercise has another effect: it can stimulate hunger. For those people who return to exercise after a considerable absence, along with those just starting to incorporate meaningful physical activity in their day-to-day lives, it is important to remind them about this fact. If healthy dietary choices are not made during these times, it will negate the weight-loss benefits the patient has just accrued. Or believing that an hour of walking entitles one to eat more than usual (which may already be more than needed) can be counterproductive.

Before the patient starts any vigorous physical activity, it is important to assess the capability of the patient regarding what is achievable for him or her. Setting unrealistic and unachievable goals is detrimental to any possible progress; worse yet, it is an "anti-motivator" because the patient may think that because he or she can't do all of these unrealistic things right away, there's no point to exercising at all.

After clinically assessing your patient, and taking into consideration his or her health history, encourage fitness activities that are varied, appealing, and can become part of their daily routine. Developing, or simply switching to, a healthy lifestyle intermittently is not going to be effective; the only way that works is to educate people about the benefits of long-term healthy behaviors and assisting them in implementing these healthy and sustainable lifestyle choices. That is what advocacy is all about.

Where Should the Patient Exercise?

The geographic location of where people live will affect the type of physical activities they do. It also will affect how often these same people partake in physical activities. No matter the setting (urban, suburban, or rural), it is imperative to recognize that each different demographic will be prone to different obstacles when it comes to exercising. For those in a primarily urban setting, there are many different ways to be physically active, as urban areas tend to have gymnasiums, community centers and other forms of group organized exercise, but that may not be true of other places, which is why this is a legitimate concern.

Even in an urban setting, there are still obstacles for some patients. For example, while there may be an abundance of possible avenues for exercise in any given city, some patients may not be in a financial position to pay related membership or access expenses in order to join a health club. Please keep this in mind, because – due to the current economic climate – you may well have patients who used to be able to afford a gym membership, but cannot anymore. However, also let patients know that certain clubs, like the YMCA, may offer subsidized or even free memberships to families in need.

Another crucial factor for many patients may be the security of where they live. Often, poorer socio-economic areas have higher rates of crime within the communities. Higher crime rates and unsafe neighborhoods (whether factual or perceived) are not conducive to regular outdoor physical activity.

In addition to the geographic "where," it is important to understand *where* the patients are coming from (figuratively speaking). If you can gain a sense of *patient perspective*, it will assist you in not only understanding why someone may have certain aversions to fitness and physical activity, but will also assist you in developing activities to overcome these barriers to physical activity and overall health behaviors.

For those patients in a rural setting, facilities such as fitness centers and gymnasiums are typically uncommon, as are community centers. Much of the physical activity of rural patients is derived from their daily routines and, therefore, instigating a change to their current routines could be necessary for the patient in order to see an increase in fitness.

A healthy lifestyle requires dedication and change regardless of where you live. Without dedication, a patient in any demographic setting will be unlikely to change his or her current eating behaviors, much less change his or her physical activity. Physically changing eating behaviors and habits, as well as increasing amounts of physical fitness, can be done almost instantly in the short term, but altering values and beliefs toward healthy living will ultimately occur over a significant period of time.

Overall, patients need to change their *perception*, which will in turn help to improve their long-term healthy behaviors. Patients need to be aware that *any* increment of physical activity will be beneficial in the long-term. Patience is needed, and assurances that body changes do not occur overnight.

In addition, patients do not need to follow strict "out of the book" line-by-line workouts for optimal results. Exercise options should be numerous and varied and will be dependent upon the individual and their current stage of fitness; as long as the exercise gets the patient moving and keeps the patient moving, that's what really counts in the long run.

Oftentimes people are overwhelmed by the specifics of exercise, and ponder questions like:

- Which muscles are targeted?
- Is the exercise anaerobic or aerobic?
- How much exercise is needed to burn how many calories?

- What is the desired heart rate?
- What is the perceived rate of exertion?
- How many repetitions and periods of rest are needed?
- What shoes are best for a specific exercise?

While these are all valid questions that can be answered throughout the course of exploring appropriate fitness programming for the individual, these questions can easily cloud the fact that almost any activity can be beneficial – even a walk around a neighborhood park, if you make the activity a habit amidst what might otherwise be a more sedentary lifestyle.

The key elements of exercise are:

- **Safety**
  - Make certain the individual is prepared with appropriate clothing: shoes are most important to avoid falling or getting an ankle injury.
- **Moderation**
  - A balance of strength training (weights, push-ups, squats, etc.) mixed with cardiovascular exercise (walking, jogging, swimming, cycling, jumping rope, etc.) will produce the best outcome. And maintain a day of rest. An overeager newcomer to fitness might over-exercise without realizing that it is better to start slowly and build endurance. Even a well-trained athlete needs a recovery day and periods of rest.
- **Variety**
  - Muscles that are exercised should have periods of rest or recovery, to avoid injury. Circuit training that targets multiple muscles can be as simple as doing 10 wall pushups, 10 squats, 20 jumping jacks, running in place for 4 minutes, and repeating this circuit again.
- **Motivation**
  - What is the motivating factor? Perhaps a weekly walk with a friend is enough motivation to get outside and walk… and this weekly walk can stimulate more activities. Maybe seeing a colleague feel more energized after a bike ride motivates one to try riding one's own bike. Or maybe a friend's illness reminds a patient of her need to maintain her own health. Any motivator, whether stemming from a good or bad situation, may be a driving force for the patient to keep in mind.

13: Fitness Plans: When, How & Why

- **Nutrition and Hydration**
  - Fitness cannot be fully successful without proper nutrition and hydration to complement the activity. Adequate hydration before, during, and after the physical activity is a MUST. The Johnny G Spinning course teaches instructors to encourage 40 ounces of water for 40 minutes of work-out (including the before, during and after exercise periods). That is the equivalent of at least three 12-ounce water bottles.
  - There are many schools of thought regarding the best ways to restore energy after a workout. Though we will not delve fully into the specifics (we are not personal trainers), many fitness programs agree that high protein, low fat foods are suggested. Even chocolate milk has been used by athletes due to the balance of protein and nutrients.

To sum up, fitness plans should be s*afe, balanced, motivating,* and combined with proper **nutrition**. There is no need for any exercise plan to become stagnant and boring. Variety in a workout plan is essential, as it's often the conduit for transitioning new healthy behaviors from what is necessary to what is meaningful and enjoyable, and thus a necessity to the patient's overall sense of well-being. Physical activity can be done inside a house, a garage, a room and even in an office space. The only catch is that your patients need to keep exercising regularly to reap the long-term rewards of exercise.

To promote a healthier and more active life, the individual should start off slowly, increase the time and intensity gradually, and choose activities they will enjoy.

Many exercise beginners, or those returning to physical activity, often make the mistake of starting out too aggressively and far too quickly. They often undertake exercises that are not suitable, are too physically strenuous and rigorous, and end up having to stop exercising in a very short period of time due to exercise-induced exhaustion or injury.

It is not uncommon for people in the initial stages of a fitness plan to become discouraged, *especially* if they have started a rigorous exercise regime. Many people believe that an aggressive workout will produce instant results. When they don't see these results within 10-14 days (or less), they are quick to dismiss regular exercise as a myth, and ineffectual.

This is why it's important for the nurse to stress the importance of low-intensity workouts for an exercise beginner. This works because the patient is far less likely to feel completely drained, or worse, get injured and stop exercising completely, due to an unrealistic and excessive fitness plan. It is important for the patient to establish fitness goals that are clear, realistic, and achievable. Low-intensity workouts, beginning with a walking plan, are the best way for reluctant individuals to start to develop new, healthy behaviors that they can transition into lifelong habits.

A combination of consistency and time (a few weeks to a few months) should allow an exercise beginner to start doing some moderate exercise. The USDA and Choosemyplate.gov give several different types of moderate exercise as examples, along with comparing these moderate activities to vigorous exercise as follows:

Moderate physical activities include:
- Walking briskly (about 3½ miles per hour)
- Bicycling (less than 10 miles per hour)
- General gardening (raking, trimming shrubs)
- Dancing
- Golf (walking and carrying clubs)
- Water aerobics
- Canoeing
- Tennis (doubles)

Vigorous physical activities include:
- Running/jogging (5 miles per hour)
- Walking very fast (4½ miles per hour)
- Bicycling (more than 10 miles per hour)
- Heavy yard work, such as chopping wood
- Swimming (freestyle laps)
- Aerobics
- Basketball (competitive)
- Tennis (singles)

In order to successfully implement long-term habits, it is essential to include different activities that are suited to the individual. While you are not necessarily the one developing the program, *per se*, ensuring that a well-rounded program is implemented is important. A mixture of cardiovascular exercise, strength training, and stretching are advised for any program at any level. Don't expect non-medical persons or non-fitness trainers to understand how to mix these all together; this will depend on the patient's goals, schedule, and fitness level, which means there are endless ways to set up any given workout program.

13: Fitness Plans: When, How & Why

Below are some basic guidelines for getting started with a complete exercise program:
- For those patients beginning a new fitness program, it is imperative to start slowly with a very basic program. People who begin a program too strenuously are unlikely to be able to sustain the program, either physically or mentally. The individual should start gradually with a very simplistic cardio routine, coupled with an introductory style of full body resistance and strength training program.
- It is essential at any stage of physical fitness to have recovery days in order to allow the body to rest and one's muscles to recuperate from the new routine.
- No matter where the person is located or if they are seeking professional fitness advice, a typical beginner program will generally include approximately **3 days of cardio activity and 2 days of strength training**. Like all exercise programs, anything is better then nothing, so if the basic program is altered either by a slight increase or decrease during the initial stages, it will still be beneficial.

Cardiovascular exercise does not need to be overly strenuous to be beneficial. People are often misinformed by the belief that one has to run miles and miles or do heavy sets of intervals in order to derive any benefit from exercise. This often misleads people into a false perception of what exercises should be done in the initial stages of a fitness program. The following cardiovascular activities are effective at all stages of programs and can be modified in their intensity as the patient becomes fitter and healthier.

Walking: Walking is a gentle, low-impact exercise that can be done just about anywhere and is therefore accessible to most patients. It doesn't require any type of technique, training, or special clothing; the only thing necessary is comfortable footwear. The impact on the body is also relatively low and therefore is far less likely to cause major injuries.

For beginners, it is easy to start in smaller increments and let the individual assess where they are, fitness-wise. By starting out slowly, people can measure their pace by time or distance. For instance, on the first walk, the individual can mark how far he can go before the walking feels strenuous; if it is 5 minutes, then the next time he walks, he should aim for 7 minutes and slowly increase from there.

The same concept applies for distance. While there are numerous high-tech gadgets that will mark time, pace, and distance, all you really need to have patients do is walk to a certain place, sign, or telegraph pole, because that way, each time they walk, their goal is to walk to something that is further away. While conceptually, it may seem overly simplistic, many people forget just how easy it can be to adapt different healthy behaviors into their current routines.

Cycling: Cycling, another low-impact cardiovascular activity, can be done almost anywhere (to what degree depends on physical health, terrain, and weather) and relatively inexpensively. If someone has never before ridden a bike, that may cause some trepidation. Older adults might be afraid of falling, and legitimately so, as balance, sight, and strength might not be what they remember; in that case, perhaps a recumbent bike, an adult tricycle, or a stationary bike would be a better option (as all offer potential exercise that is greatly beneficial).

Like walking, the inception of a cycling program starts with the ability of the patient; it may take some time to gain confidence and to ride for a prolonged period of time; after that, the individual marks progress by either time or distance.

Cycling has numerous benefits and provides a great cardiovascular workout as well as strength training, with little risk of over-use or strain. It's relatively cheap; once you have a bike and related safety equipment, all that is necessary is to start biking around the neighborhood. Bicycle riding can also be a wonderful social outlet, if one finds a friend or partner with whom to ride. (Otherwise, it's potentially a nice solo adventure and time alone.)

Programs like Johnny G's Spinning© programs by Madd Dog Athletics have movies and stationary bikes for sale. And many gyms and YMCAs offer frequent cycling classes.

> **Debbie's note:** As veteran cyclist and instructor for the YMCA for six years, I have enjoyed teaching people of all ages, from 14 through the mid-80s. I strongly encourages this activity.

Cycling in a group exercise class offers companionship and support, with a trained instructor who can help troubleshoot cycling with any medical issues or special concerns. Overcoming the potential intimidation of riding a stationary bike in a dark room with loud music can ultimately rejuvenate and inspire people to ride on!

Swimming: Water-based exercise in any form is advantageous for people at any stage of exercise, from beginner through to advanced levels. Swimming is often overlooked for many reasons, most notably the need to wear a bathing suit and the requirement to find a pool. Although not technically as easy to access as bike riding or walking, swimming boasts the same advantages with one distinct extra, the lack of stress on joints. Swimming also provides a full body workout of all muscles without the strain that can be induced by other exercises.

While many people are hesitant about swimming, individuals need to know that it's not just about technique and looking good in the water. There are classes that can be taken, such as water aerobics, pool jogging, and kicking, all of which have outstanding health benefits. Swimming is often encouraged for overweight individuals and older individuals, as the lack of stress and strain on joints and muscle tissue make the recovery time from swimming minimal. Remember, though, that the resistance of working out in water can be great, and might not be well suited to everyone's needs. Even a little self-experimentation in a pool can help determine what feels comfortable, before one decides whether or not water exercise is the right choice. Start with knee raises, repeating 10 times on both sides, can be a good beginning program. Cardiovascular activity is also important in any healthy lifestyle, even when swimming, and a mixture of activities is preferable to avoid boredom and to get the body's muscles and joints involved in a combination of different movements. Therefore, your patient can incorporate cardio-exercise in the pool by including jogging for a few minutes in between leg exercises. Encouraging any continuous and safe movement is a good start, and can minimize fear of falling (of course, other safety measures to avoid drowning must be observed).

Strength Training: In conjunction with cardio fitness, it is essential to incorporate full body strength and resistance training. Weight-bearing exercise can reduce bone loss, especially in women when the need for calcium is high. Strength training has a multitude of benefits such as increasing strength, joint flexibility, weight loss and increased muscle tone (Braith et al, 2006).

As with a cardio-based routine, it is important to integrate strength training gradually to avoid injury and overuse stress. Images of sculpted bodies lifting large weights often dissuade individuals from pursuing any form or style of weight training, which is why it's important to convey to the patient that large, cumbersome weights are not the answer.

Depending on the patient's age, stage, ability, and environment, strength training can be adapted to fit almost any need. For children, something as simple as a jumping program can improve bone mineral density (MacKelvie, et. al., 2002). A seven-month jumping intervention program among prepubescent Asian and white boys showed there was increased bone accrual for boys of average or low BMI, but accrual was not detected among boys with high BMI. Weight-bearing exercises (even in boys) should be emphasized early, before weight gain, to promote optimal growth and to emphasize healthy habits.

> **NOTE:** Throughout the lifespan, there remain differences between the effects of weight bearing or strength exercises on males and females. The focus tends to be on women, either at risk of osteoporosis, or those who already have osteoporosis (providing they can exercise at all).

While most people do not routinely go to a gym, strength training can be done to a minimal extent at home, which will still improve health. Some at-home exercises include push ups (knee-based or against a wall to begin), triceps and shoulder exercises and biceps curls; all of these can be done without any additional weights being added.

If the individual is adamant on incorporating weights, small ones (approximately 3-5 pounds for women, and 5-10 pounds for men) are ideal. While, for many, the weights will seem too light, repetition is the key; for those who have not been physically active for some time, 15-20 repetitions of a single exercise with this level of weight will be significant.

It is important that different muscle groups are worked. If the individual is unsure of the correct technique or types of exercise, you should encourage them to pursue more information through literature on the Internet (which has literally thousands of articles), fitness magazines and, where appropriate, the patient should consult a local gym (as many places will do an introduction to weights and machines completely free of charge).

When your patient starts this type of exercise, you should go through whatever incorporated plans and routines the patient has come up with in order to ensure that he is incorporating a mixture of exercises, as well as taking appropriate rest days in between to avoid over-use injuries. This does not include writing a full-fledged fitness plan for the patient, as you are not a personal trainer; instead, ask your patient what he's doing and how, as that should give you enough information to figure out whether the patient really does know what he's doing.

Summary

Overall, The HERO Guide to Health advocates that exercise in many shapes and forms can be beneficial. Supporting your patient to help develop and incorporate a fitness routine that can be maintained over time is essential to successfully promote healthy living. Helping to set realistic and balanced exercise plans can alleviate your patient's confusion and frustration when starting new exercise programs.

"Demystifying" exercise myths may be the best thing medical professionals can do to help an exercise beginner, as many patients have no idea what constitutes real exercise, how the body benefits from it, and how therapeutic moderate or vigorous exercise can improve endurance, health, and self-esteem over time.

Patients should choose a variety of activities, as that's the best way to keep from being bored. They also should be guided to understand what is achievable for a beginner (as well as what isn't), in order to avoid exercise-induced injuries.

Through education and empowerment, obesity and its ill effects can be reversed over time and with dedication. As a medical professional, you must aim to educate and instill the idea that it is important that people adapt healthy activity behaviors in conjunction with healthy eating behaviors.

When people are educated, they, in turn, have the power of choice. When they choose to make healthy and educated decisions because they understand that is what's in their long-term best interest, that is what constitutes true health advocacy.

References

Braith, R.W, and Stewart, K.J. (2006). Resistance Exercise Training Its Role in the Prevention of Cardiovascular Disease. Retrieved 05/12/12 from the American Heart Association Website at http://circ.ahajournals.org/content/113/22/2642.extract?sid=cefeabf6-9b4a-4178-9138-73663fe69022

Centers for Disease Control (CDC), (2012), Physical Activity for Everyone. Retrieved on 06/07/12 at http://www.cdc.gov/physicalactivity/everyone/health/index.html

Mackelvie, K.J., McKay, H.A., Khan, K.M. and Crocker, P.R.E. (2001) A school-based exercise intervention augments bone mineral accrual in early pubertal girls. *Journal of Pediatrics*. 139, 501–508.

Otto, M., and Smits, J. (2011) *Exercise for Mood and Anxiety: Proven Strategies for Overcoming Depression and Enhancing Well-Being*. Oxford University Press US.

Poirier, P. and Després, J.P. (2001) Exercise in weight management of obesity. *Cardiol Clin*. 2001 Aug;19 (3):459-70. Retrieved 06/06/12 from http://www.ncbi.nlm.nih.gov/pubmed/11570117

Chapter 14
Health Advocacy: How to BE Your Own HERO©

"Our bodies are our gardens – our wills are our gardeners"
— *William Shakespeare*

    Throughout this guide, we have reinforced the idea that obesity can be prevented and/or reversed. Through a combination of health advocacy and education, people can learn *how* to make better choices, and understand *why* doing so is the best option. As a healthcare professional, you can empower people to be their own health advocates through education, positive reinforcement and, perhaps the most important thing of all, by being honest, yet nonjudgmental.

    In the same way that every person has his own genetic physical predispositions to shape and structural development, each patient referred to you will have very different values, priorities, and beliefs. In many cases, none of these will take on a medical construct and, therefore, as the health provider, it is imperative for you to simultaneously assess behavioral traits that heighten the risk of obesity. As healthcare providers, it is important to recognize that we should not only approach medicine from a symptomatic perspective, but equally important, to approach preventive healthcare with educating patients at the forefront of our minds.

> ## Chapter 14 Objectives:
> 1. Identify human drives that affect health behavior and the potential for change
> 2. Explain the need for nurses to continue health promotion efforts
> 3. Determine how to facilitate a patient's change in health behaviors through education and patience

14: Health Advocacy: How to Be Your Own HERO©

We at the HERO Program believe that patients need to be empowered in order to make changes to their current lifestyles. They need encouragement and education, otherwise they'll never be able to "be (their) own HERO©" as our motto states. Fortunately, healthcare professionals – especially nurses – are well situated to give this encouragement and education at any age.

People look to nurses not only for medical care, but also for support of their overall health and well being. As nurses, health education for our patients is the best tool we can arm them with regarding their own health advocacy once they step away from the clinical setting.

One caveat, though: depending on the setting and reason for a patient visit, any given nurse may see a patient only once. For such nurses, advocacy will be a much more difficult, if not impossible, task. Other times, though, nurses have the opportunity to build rapport through continued visits.

Either way, do not underestimate the impact of a nurse on the patient. Demonstrating knowledge of health and helping provide people with the right educational tools can ultimately help them improve their health and health environment. By helping our patients understand that the nurse is a medical professional who does not just treat, but also provides health advice, resources, and a broad human perspective, we can ultimately encourage patients to want to learn more, advocate, and take charge of their own bodies.

As well-trained nurses, we easily forget how things that may seem trivial to us might be foreign to a patient. Therefore, patience and clear explanations should be given for medical terms and advice.

Societal attitudes towards weight, body type and what is attractive continue to suggest that everyone should aspire to a thin body type. This does not help patients to sustain weight loss; instead, this only causes patients to feel more insecure regarding their own struggles. In addition, due perhaps to the myriad of media avenues, society more often than not falsely categorizes those who do not fit into the "thin" category as lazy or self-destructive, which can be misleading at the absolute best.

While the causes of obesity, more often than not, stem from a lack of basic nutrition and fitness education, the wide promotion of "quick-fix" schemes and pharmaceuticals continues to be broadcast as the underlying solution for obesity. There are pills, shakes, meal plans, routines, machines – all are hailed as *the answers* to obesity, when it is clear that, in most incidences, obesity can be overcome and/or prevented through *education*.

If education isn't given, no scheme or diet in the world will keep weight off, nor will it improve health. This is why we need to consider many different questions when attempting to help our patients, including the following:

1. **What foods do they eat?**
   Adults make choices every time they head to the grocery store, but most focus on the price of the food rather than on their own health. In addition, many people are under the false impression that to eat healthy, you have to eat expensively, but this is not true. (Many fresh vegetables are the same price as the canned options.)

   Some people don't realize that they may save money by buying fresh produce in its original form. For example, whole apples, lettuce, and carrots are often a fraction of the cost of their washed and packaged counterparts. Remember – what food patients tend to eat comes down to *choice* and choice can be mitigated by good nutritional education.

2. **Do they have access to and/or interest in health and activity?**
   Access is often proclaimed to be a strong determining factor of obesity. In this case, is there *access* to healthy foods?

   Usually, if people can access McDonalds®, KFC® or Taco Bell®, then it is safe to assume that there is access to a supermarket or corner store. The patient must make the choice to *utilize* these options, which takes more effort than driving through a fast food restaurant, but the *access* is always there.

   In a case where someone is willing to utilize a fast food restaurant but not a grocery store, it is the *interest* that is lacking, specifically, the interest in purchasing and preparing healthy foods.

   Educating people about the positive effects of eating healthy can lead to an increased awareness of healthy foods, as well as the access they currently have. Most importantly, it empowers people to make better choices.

   The second part of the question would be, "Is there access to physical activity?" This is often answered as "no" when it might be a "yes" instead, mostly because people mistakenly associate access to physical activity as access to a large multi-purpose gymnasium. These can be expensive, and might not be located in convenient settings for many of the patients you will see.

   The key, again, is *education*. People should not rely upon expensive gyms or country club-type settings in order to get their daily physical activity. Simple solutions, such as taking the stairs instead of an elevator, taking pets for their needed walks, walks with family and/or co-workers, and some indoor activities, all constitute *daily physical activity*. For patients, the lesson lies within *making* the time for exercise and utilizing what they have.

14: Health Advocacy: How to Be Your Own HERO©

Overcoming an aversion to physical activity while igniting an interest is critical. As a health educator, you can utilize evidence-based research provided by the U.S. Department of Health and Human Services at www.health.gov on the benefits of physical activity that include, but are not limited to, reduced blood pressure, the potential lowering of cholesterol, and more.

When providing health services to families, you will often find that children are more likely to be open to change and learning new behaviors than their parents. In many instances, parents might perceive a recommended change in behaviors as a judgment of their parenting techniques or disapproval by you, the medical professional. This can result in defensive behavior which will hinder attempts to assist the patient. Therefore, taking a nonjudgmental tone is best.

Each individual you see will have different perceptions and ideas on how to approach obesity, including the fact that some people won't even care. As a health advocate, promoter, and educator, this last attitude can be frustrating. Just remember that each individual is motivated by both intrinsic and extrinsic factors. The small amount of time you have with them means that you need to make the most of it.

Simple suggestions that are non-judgmental and aren't condescending to the patient are critical. No matter what the person's situation, background, or social status, you need to remove any personal bias and address the actual issue at hand. This is not an easy task.

Ultimately, the role you want to take is one of *facilitation*. While it may be blatantly obvious to you that a full transformation and revitalization is in the best interest of the family, the parents need to come to that conclusion themselves, albeit with some subtle guidance from you. It is in this instance that you, as a healthcare professional, also become an educator and promoter of the benefits of health education.

Your ability to reverse obesity trends lies in your *approach* to the patient. Ensuring you keep a balanced and positive outlook from the beginning will assist you in overcoming obstacles that people will often put forward. It is through precise and succinct questions that you will be able to get to the core of unhealthy eating and behaviors, which will help to overcome these obstacles much more easily.

The most common of these obstacles in overweight adults, and adults with overweight children, tend to come in the form of the following statements:

"*I'm too busy,*" or
"*I ate a high fat diet and wasn't overweight as a child,*" or

"Society encourages poor eating choices," or
"Eating healthy is expensive."

Some good answers to those questions follow:

"I'm too busy:" This is by far the most common excuse. Yes, schedules are busy, but if something is a priority, one will make time for it. So make time for exercise.

Exercise doesn't need to take an hour, as just 30 minutes a day is effective. Basic strategies such as walking around the neighborhood, taking the stairs (if physically able), or parking further away are all simple, yet positive, strategies toward healthy behaviors. Time to exercise doesn't need to consume hours of the day. Having a plan to exercise and regularly scheduling exercise can become part of any routine.

"I ate a high fat diet and wasn't overweight as a child:" We all know that dieting has become popular over the past thirty years. As technological advances decrease the requirement for physical labor, people are going to put on weight if they do not counter the loss of daily physical activity, which is the main reason for this phenomenon. Saying this in a matter-of-fact way may be enough to get past anyone's initial defensiveness.

Of course, when parents are questioned about their children's eating habits, they will often become defensive very quickly, as they see such questioning as direct criticism of their parenting techniques. At any stage of obesity, but especially *childhood obesity*, it is important to align with the parents and educate rather than judge.

In this case, you can perhaps defuse any defensiveness by *agreeing* with them. Yes, they most likely did eat a high fat diet as a child but, comparatively, there were fewer processed foods and they exercised more. (When discussing exercise, you need to let them know that you are *not* referring to time at a gym; this exercise was simply walking to school, playing outside, not having computer games, riding bikes to go anywhere, and so on.) Highlighting these differences is a good segue into encouraging families to do more things, together, outside.

"Society encourages poor eating choices:" With so many quick, easy and cheap choices, societal changes toward eating habits and the contradiction television portrays confuses many individuals. On one hand, the media delivers scenes of delicious, cheap, high-calorie and nutritionally worthless food, but on the other, it encourages and endorses the perpetually thin body type. People are confused by these contradictions, and in many instances will *not* understand the amount of calories in their favorite convenience foods. Pointing out that a Big Mac®, say, has more calories than a hamburger cooked at home might be the first way to get through to them.

"I can't exercise... I'm too old and/or fat:" Many people you will assess and see have been overweight or obese for a significant amount of time. As with age, being overweight is not an excuse for not exercising. Educating the patient on beginning a healthy eating and exercise routine is important. In the process, you must make it very clear that success will not be quick or easy. Exercise will take dedication and time, but the results will be worth it.

Of course, there is no point in the patient immediately attempting to run four miles if he or she has lived a sedentary life to this point, nor is cutting out all of the unhealthy foods he or she eats daily. The inception of healthy behaviors should be *gradual* and goals need to be *achievable*. People need to start walking, swimming, biking, or engaging in other exercises that don't involve a lot of friction and or strain on the body and are perfect for beginners (r*efer back to Chapter 9 for more information*).

Finally, as exercise education and nutritional education *complement* one another, people need to understand that exercising more doesn't mean that they can eat more as a reward. While this would be great in theory, it doesn't work in practice.

"Eating healthy is expensive:" Quantity over quality occurs all too often when talking about nutrition. People often think that, to eat healthy, food has to be expensive, while food preparation must be time consuming. Like all matters concerning nutrition, education is paramount toward reversing this mistaken belief. Shopping smart, and looking for fresh produce, eggs, dairy and whole wheat options are simply smarter choices, and are not necessarily more expensive.

The most important thing to remember is that an honest approach to obesity is essential. In earlier chapters, diagnostic techniques and physical examination techniques were discussed in a very clinical manner, which is unlikely to help a patient who's never been exposed to clinical language of this nature before. This is why, when communicating to patients the adverse effects directly linked to obesity, it is important to conceptualize and explain in detail at the level the patient is going to be most able to understand. Some of the questions you can help resolve are the following:

- What is high cholesterol and what does it do to the body?
- How can it be reversed?
- What simple changes can be made to prevent it?

The same approach should be used with diabetes, heart disease, and other, obesity-related adverse health conditions. As the people you are likely to see come from all different backgrounds, cultures, and have different levels of education, a "one size fits all" mentality is not likely to work. This is why explaining clinical concepts at a basic level is important.

People need to understand what happens to the body when it is not looked after, which is why your role as an educator is vital.

Unlike many health concerns, obesity is one that is visible, and rarely is a medical procedure required to diagnose obesity. Openly and honestly discussing obesity and the fact that it is choice-related (that being the choice of what to eat, and the choice of what activity to partake in) often is motivation enough for people to want to change their habits.

While people may wish to change their behavior in the short-term, they may not realize that the only changes that are effective are those that are instituted, and followed, on a long-term basis. With so many quick fixes available to people, it is very important to explain long-term strategies and preventative health concepts, as they are the only proven way to keep weight off and maintain health over time. People will always look for, search for and pay for a "quick fix," but empirical data shows that dramatic weight loss in a short period of time is *not sustainable in the long-term*. Knowledge of this should help you, as a nurse, to be better able to give good guidance to patients.

Understanding what drives and motivates people in both the long and short term is essential in health education and obesity prevention. Knowing the core drivers and motivators of your patient allows you to instill the promotion of healthy lifestyle choices, healthy behaviors, and a heightened level of self-esteem on an individual basis. By educating, we can empower. By empowering, we assist in getting people to make the right choices and decisions, which can be a lifelong lesson.

People are driven by numerous factors, some of which are easier to access and transform then others. The outline below gives some insight into what drives and motivates people on a day to day basis, providing an overview on how people make decisions. By starting with behaviors, you can filter in ways to address and encourage people to transform their actions. You can't expect to change values and beliefs in a short period of time, because you need to establish strategies with each individual patient in order to ensure longevity and success. But long-term behaviors can be changed, especially if a gradual approach is taken.

Behaviors

Changing certain behaviors and habits is where you can have the most impact. **Behavior** is defined as the actions or reactions of a person in response to external or internal stimuli. Transforming eating habits, encouraging exercise, and changing fitness and nutrition behaviors are the first steps. Once behaviors are changed, you can then develop a greater understanding of why the changes have been made through education.

Education

By failing to educate people, we fail to advocate choice, and in not promoting choice, we are restricting patients from the outset. The job of a primary healthcare professional is not only to *treat* patients, but, just as importantly, to *educate* them. Whether treating or assessing individuals or families, education is fundamental in getting people to adjust their behaviors.

Beliefs

Beliefs are not developed in the short term, as they are opinions or convictions in which an individual holds a proposition or premise to be true. Remember that you are not going to change beliefs automatically: no matter how much conviction you have or what you say, it's often going to be met with excuses and/or retorts to the contrary. Beliefs have been established *over time*, so in order to change them, it will take continued education and behavioral changes before beliefs will be affected.

Values

Values are established in early childhood, and are usually passed on through generations. When attending to children, with or without a parent present, it is important to espouse healthy behaviors, educate all parties, and begin to transform their beliefs and attitudes toward living healthy.

After addressing intrinsic factors, it is important to understand those extrinsic factors that can lead to obesity. Those confronted daily with weight issues often blame the increase of their weight on external factors. People often use food to console themselves in times of emotional, economic, and psychological times of hardship. (It is rare for people to turn to healthy foods, such as fruits or vegetables, during such times.) Thus, the notion of "comfort food" is derived from sugary, high fat and high caloric choices. Also be aware that people dealing with anxiety and depression often lose the motivation to partake in any physical activity whatsoever, which just exacerbates any poor food choices they may make; the combination of poor diet choices and a sedentary lifestyle invariably results in weight gain.

Holding people accountable for their lifestyle choices and health behaviors is essential in combating the obesity epidemic that is plaguing the U.S. Not surprisingly, the burden of healthcare costs is in the billions of dollars for obesity-related healthcare, and hospitalizations due to diabetes, heart disease, asthma, and stroke – even in children. That's why "calling" patients on their behavior in a nonjudgmental way is so important, as it may be the only way you have to get through to certain patients.

Obesity is a very sensitive subject. There is a myriad of conflicting literature on underlying causes and precursors that are widely discussed, debated and reported on. Some medical professionals suggest that obesity is genetic in nature, which in essence dissolves the majority of responsibility from the patient by claiming that obesity is not within the individual's day-to-day control. This is a very dangerous view to pass on to a patient suffering from obesity, as it abrogates any sense of individual responsibility.

Rather than removing responsibility from the individual, healthcare professionals should encourage people to do whatever they can to improve their health. Patients must become empowered, take whatever responsibility they can, and advocate for their own health and wellbeing.

Overcoming obesity will not be easy for most patients. Committing to a healthy lifestyle, along with harnessing healthy behaviors, is the only proven, long-term solution. And perhaps by the already-overweight or obese patient taking action *now*, he or she may be able to pass healthier behavior patterns to the next generation *later*; such is the power of prevention. In so doing, your patient will have become his or her very own HERO.

Appendix A: SOAP Notes

Date:		
Patient Name:		
Referred by:		
Date of Birth:	Race:	Ethnicity:
Height:	Weight:	Cholesterol:
BMI:	Blood Pressure:	Blood Glucose:

Health History:	Check all that apply:	Describe below:
Diabetes (Type 1 or 2)		
Heart disease/		
High blood pressure		
Arthritis/Joint pain		
Blood disorder		
Vision disturbance		
Physical disability		

SUBJECTIVE: Patient is a _____year-old male/female with a history of _____who complains of _____ which began_____days/months/years ago. Pt. complains of _____, _____, and _____

Typical Diet:_____ Activities:_____
Frequency:_____

OBJECTIVE: BP:_____/_____.
Labs include: _____

Physical Exam:	Describe Abnormalities
Head/Eyes/Ears/Nose/Throat:	
Heart/Vascular:	
Lungs/Chest:	
Abdomen/Digestive:	
Musculoskeletal/Extremities:	
Neurological:	

(Continued)

Appendix A: SOAP Notes

ASSESSMENT: Pt. is a _____ year-old with a history of _____ and current complaints of_____
_____

Based on report of_____and objective data including: _____, patient is at risk of _____
_____

PLAN: Return for follow-up in _____days/months.

Recommendations: Patient increases intake of_____,
_____, and _____.

Reduce intake of _____ & _____(ex: chips and sugared cereals). Increase activity and fitness by adding 15/30/45 minutes of daily/weekly activities like: _____, _____, _____

Referral to:_____

Phone:_____

Appendix B: Obesity 101

The Nurse Should Educate the Patient to:
- **Understand risk factors**
    - Obesity raises the risk of heart disease, stroke, hypertension, high cholesterol, osteoarthritis, gallstones and more
    - Do you already have risk factors for heart disease and stroke?
    - Are you a smoker? Do you have a family history of diabetes, heart disease or stroke?
- **Pay attention to your behaviors**
    - Keep a sleep diary
    - Keep an exercise diary
    - Keep a food diary
- **Share feelings with a friend or family member**
    - Start talking about changes you want to make. The first step is to let go of denial and recognize that you can make changes
- **Follow-up with your nurse or doctor**
    - Do you need referrals to a dietician or diabetes consultant
    - Do you have a doctor you feel comfortable with?
- **Learn how to substitute.** Slow and steady changes work best. An *all* or *nothing* attitude will not last long, but small steps can.
    - Substitute: drink diet soda instead of sugared soda; use a smaller cup for sugared drinks. OR, better yet, drink water instead – and use a LARGE cup for water to encourage more intake
    - Take the stairs at work every other day instead of elevator (if you are able) OR take a 15-minute break to walk (indoors or out)
    - Go to sleep 30 minutes earlier
    - Watch 30 minutes less of TV a day
    - Take one slice of bread off the burger or sandwich

Appendix C: HERO Recipe for Success

TEN STEPS for the HERO Recipe for SUCCESS

1. Select *one* choice for each of three meals daily from the HERO MENU. Over time, you will learn to make slight menu changes successfully
2. Try this plan for *at least* a week (the goal is not weight loss, the goal is modifying eating habits, which, in turn, can lead to weight loss). Realistically, successful weight loss can take at least 3 months, if done healthfully
3. Follow this plan at home *AND* at a restaurant
4. If you are eating out, choose the menu item that *best resembles* the HERO menu
5. Ask for *substitutions*, if possible (ask for grilled instead of fried...)
6. Breakfast, lunch, and dinner items are i*nterchangeable* (i.e., breakfast for dinner)
7. The goal is <500 calories per meal (some restaurants now have such choices)
8. Drink WATER before, during, and after meals
9. The goal is NOT to *starve* your body! Reducing calories (since many of us eat more calories than our bodies need) can help lose weight and maintain a healthy weight. Balance of eating fewer calories, but eating more fiber and protein to feel more full is key!
10. Learn to eat to live, not live to eat!

The above steps illustrates the importance of three meals a day, but most people enjoy a few snacks in between. Snacking does not necessarily mean overeating. In fact, many "diets" encourage snacking, but the challenge is to choose healthy, low calorie snacks. The downfall of snacking is that the foods selected are often eaten by the handful, and thus there is no portion control. While a handful of roasted almonds (10 or so nuts) can make a good snack that is high in protein, the ease with which people take a second and third handful can turn a good snack into a high calorie, high fat overindulgence. Let's keep in mind the goal of the snack when we eat it. Think about the driving force for your snacking:

- **Because you are hungry**
    - When you first change your eating pattern, you will likely feel more hungry. Drink water and eat a high protein, high fiber, low-

fat snack. Good options are a slice of whole grain toast with peanut butter or a glass of low-fat milk.

- **Because you have a habit of eating**
  - This is the most difficult type of snacking to curb, since we must shift a behavior. The goal here is to be able to snack, but replace your snacks with low calorie options, and monitor the portions. A low calorie yogurt or a banana, or even drinking a cup of tea, can fill the need while not increasing calorie intake too much.
- **Because you have low blood sugar**
  - Many diets do recommend the maintenance of steady blood sugar rates throughout the day and, therefore, recommend eating up to 6 small meals a day. Complex carbohydrates (rather than a simple sugar like chocolate, cookies, etc.) like whole grain toast make a good choice.

Depending on the reason for your snacking, you can make the best choices.

And remember that ***portion control*** is essential! Always place your snack on a plate or in a bowl before starting to nibble, otherwise it is far too tempting to keep eating from the bag. Here are a few examples of simple snacks.

Low calorie:

- Limit snacks to <100 calories per snack (up to 2 snacks a day)
  - Cup of strawberries or blueberries
  - ½ cup of low-fat cottage cheese with a tomato
  - Banana and ½ cup of milk
  - Non-fat small cappuccino (no added syrups or sugar)
  - Low-fat string cheese and an apple
  - Low-fat, low calorie yogurt (check sugar content – <10g sugar is best)
  - Sugar-free pudding snack (for a portion-controlled sweet treat)
  - Frozen fudge bar (for a portion-controlled sweet snack)

High Fiber:

- Limit snacks to <150 calories
  - Slice of whole grain toast with tsp. of peanut butter
  - Peach and ½ cup of plain yogurt
  - ½ cup plain oatmeal with raisins
  - Small handful of dry roasted almonds

- 6-7 whole grain crackers with celery and peanut or almond butter

Because so many Americans have become accustomed to eating out so frequently, many of us have forgotten how to eat at home, or how to eat *well* outside our home. The goal of HERO is to empower you to make *simple changes*, and to eat a variety of fresh healthful foods. The HERO MENU is provided as a TOOL to guide your healthy choices. With thousands of cookbooks, recipes, and health diets available, choices are overwhelming and confusing. This menu is designed to highlight a GENERAL visualization of how we should be eating on a daily basis.

What are the essential components of daily food that we need to keep in mind?

CALORIC INTAKE/PORTION SIZE: many Americans eat far *too many calories* – and often do not realize this. *Portions* are excessively large (especially at restaurants), and we snack *too often* and *too much.*

FAT CONTENT: While it is recommended that 25-35% of calories be from fat, this includes the healthy fat from foods like avocado and nuts. Only 10% of our food intake should be from *saturated fat*. This means that we should take in only 22 grams of saturated fat for a typical 2,000-calorie diet. Unfortunately, when we eat out, most of the fat is saturated fat! So, make the best choice possible to limit your total fat. Many restaurants now have nutritional information onsite or online. There is a wide variation of fat content in foods, and just a bit of legwork on your part can enable you to eat out more successfully and healthfully. Even at a food venue that has relatively better choices, there is still a wide variety of how well you can eat.

For example: choosing a 6" meatball pepperoni melt at Subway® adds 29 grams of fat, whereas a 6" B.L.T. is only 9 grams of fat and, better yet, the 6" Turkey Breast has **3.5** grams of fat! What should you pick?? Remember, though, that adding cheese and condiments like dressing and mayonnaise, also adds more fat (Subway, 2012).

SALT/SODIUM INTAKE: Our taste buds have become accustomed to the salty foods we eat at restaurants and in prepared foods. Cooking at home is a good way to slowly reinvent our taste buds by preparing fresh foods that require little salt. Beginning to appreciate the natural flavors of foods and adding unsalted condiments can reduce sodium intake. Use salsa, hot sauce, pepper, lemon or lime juice, and herbs to add flavor without adding too much salt.

Appendix C: HERO Recipe for Success

VARIETY: A plate with a variety of colors and flavors is more exciting and inviting. Again, the overriding flavor is *salty*!

NUTRIENTS: Which vitamins and minerals are in our meals? How can we make better choices to include more nutrients? Choose: fresh instead of fried vegetables; steamed instead of canned vegetables; squash instead of white potatoes; grilled beef instead of hot dogs, etc.

ALCOHOL: *(**Disclaimer:** Though HERO does not recommend alcohol consumption, we recognize that many people DO consume alcohol. So, make the best choice possible and drink responsibly)*

There remains controversial research regarding the heart benefits of alcohol consumption versus the risks of accidental injury, mortality and chronic disease. There are currently no true recommendations advocating consumption of alcohol, though some sources indicate that one serving a day for women, and two servings a day for men, might offer some heart benefits without the risk. Remember, though, that a serving is classified as:

- One 5 oz. glass of wine
- One 12 oz. low calorie beer
- 1 ½ oz. of spirits

(Cleveland Clinic, 2012).

Remember that the caloric intake of any beverage (especially alcoholic beverages with fruit juices and mixers) can increase empty calorie consumptions (plus the dehydrating effects of alcohol). Also remember that, for people with a health history of diabetes, liver or kidney conditions, history of familial alcohol addiction, etc., the risks might outweigh any benefit. Consultation with a doctor before initiating alcohol consumption is highly recommended for everyone.

Perhaps due to the relative affordability, convenience, and expectation of fast food and fast service, we have forgotten how simple it can be to eat even better at home. While shopping for and preparing foods at home seems eternally time-consuming and a chore to most, in reality, the process can take less time than the driving to a restaurant, waiting to be seated, waiting to order and receive our food, and driving home.

Eating has become a national pastime in this country, and that is the essence of the obesity culture. We have forgotten why we eat. Americans are eating now mainly for pleasure, and not for health and nutrition. When we step back and recognize this, we can begin to modify how we eat. Not to say that eating should not be pleasant and fun, but the fanfare of eating out does not need to occur daily.

We must always keep in mind the nutrient value (or lack thereof) of what we ingest.

- Does it have protein? If so, is it lean? Can we make a better choice? Opt for grilled over fried, skinless over breaded, etc.
- Does it have fiber? The more refined and processed an item is, the less fiber it has. White bread lacks the fiber that whole wheat or seeded bread has. Can we make a better choice? Choose brown over white, grainy over smooth.
- Does it have dark leafy greens? When we do eat salads, does it have dark greens or is it all pale iceberg lettuce? The darker the better, and more loaded with vitamins and minerals.

HERO developed a simple Menu and Fitness Plans *(see Appendices D & E)* for you to visualize and select meals and activities that can work for your patients. Helping explain the simplicity and common theme of all successful plans can help jump-start your patient to begin a new pattern of health!

With the many name-brand diets programs available, it can be overwhelming to select an appropriate plan. Our goal is to summarize and show you and your patients the common themes among them that can lead to successful healthy eating patterns, which can ultimately lead to weight loss as well. Helping patients understand that there is no *single* diet plan that is best,

References

Cleveland Clinic. (2012). Retrieved on 05/06/12 at http://my.clevelandclinic.org/heart/disorders/alcoholandheartdisease.aspx

Subway (2012). Retrieved on 05/04/12 at http://www.subway.com/nutrition/nutritionlist.aspx

Appendix D: HERO Fitness Plan

Date: _____

Name: _____ Exercise Partner: _____

Current Weight: _____ BMI: _____
Desired Weight: _____ BMI: _____
Realistic Weight: TBD

Goals: Circle all that apply & describe:
1. **General health:** _____
2. **Weight loss:** _____
3. **Strength:** _____
4. **Medical Condition:** _____
5. **Social:** _____
6. **Other:** _____

Favorite Activities:
1. _____
2. _____
3. _____

What activities would you or could you realistically fit in to your schedule?
Light Activity: such as walking, grocery shopping (parking in far spot)
   1. _____   2. _____   3. _____
Moderate Activity: such as dancing, general gardening, touring bicycle riding,
   1. _____   2. _____   3. _____
Rigorous Activity: such as fast walking, tennis (singles), jogging, basketball (competitive), climbing multiple flights of steps

Week 1: commit 20 minutes a day
Week 2: commit 30 minutes a day

Sunday	Monday	Tuesday	Wednesday	Thursday	Friday	Saturday
Rest Focus on light activity	20/30 minutes walking indoors or out	20/30 minutes climbing steps or stepping high in place	20/30 minutes bike riding, or fast walking indoors or out	20/30 minutes gardening or moderate house work	20/30 minutes fast walking or jogging	Rest Focus on light activity

My below signature is to acknowledge for *myself* that I will plan, commit, sweat, drink water and prioritize my exercise routine.

X_____

Appendix D: HERO Fitness Plan

> **Note: *How to Succeed With a HERO Fitness Plan***
>
> Granted, the hardest part of beginning any fitness programming is the first start! How can we encourage our patients to initiate a plan they have never done before? Remember that, as nurses, we often introduce new habits and self-care for patients. When we care for patients in a hospital setting, we often provide specific teaching for many conditions. We may teach how to change wound dressings, how to give self-injections, or how to transfer from bed to wheelchair after surgery, etc. For a post-surgical patient, it is the nurse or nursing assistant who facilitates and helps the patient sit up, walk to the bathroom, then walk down the hall. We encourage ambulation post-operatively to help with the rehabilitation post-surgery. Ambulation is needed to improve circulation, reduce the risk of blood clots, reduce the risk of pneumonia, etc. Just as our role involves activity in the hospital, we can equally offer a few words of encouragement and even a sample plan for our patients beyond their hospital stay.
>
> Sometimes, hearing a plan from a nurse face-to-face can be more effective than seeing a plan in writing, or watching a weight loss program. So, even taking a few moments to discuss the patient's daily routine, and how to schedule time for even a little acitivity can be very helpful to jump-start a new fitness schedule.
>
> The HERO Fitness Plan is intended only as a guide to show how easily fitness can be implemented, with or without a gym membership. Many people do not think of walking as "exercise" that can be an effective way to start a good habit of activity. For patients first initiating activity, they should understand how light exercise can be effective. The goal is to ultimately shift from light exercise to moderate and vigourous exercise 5 days a week.

In a Nutshell – Helping Patients Learn How to:

- Get started. Always start *today* and not tomorrow!
- Find a friend, neighbor, or family member to accompany you
- Hold yourself accountable… staying healthy is for you!
- Focus on your positives!
    - Pat yourself on the back for starting and getting activated!
    - Take a moment to look at yourself in the mirror and tell yourself "I can and I will do it!"
- Wear appropriate clothing
    - Gym shoes
    - Breathable clothing
- Drink water before, during, and after exercise
- Reward yourself with a new workout shirt, not with food!

Appendix E: HERO Menu

HERO Menu

Take the first step for your better health. Chose one menu from each category. Your challenge: Make or find similar items and enjoy them!

Breakfast: — *Calories:*

#1 **Whole Grain Cereal and Milk** – ½ cup non-fat or low-fat milk. 1 cup unsweetened grain cereal *like Kashi*®, *Oatmeal squares*, *Wheeties*®…& banana — *<500*

#2 **Eggs and Toast** – 1 or 2 eggs your way; 1 or 2 slices whole grain toast & banana — *<500*

#3 **Yogurt and Fruit** – low-fat/non-fat yogurt with fruit cup (berries, banana, cantaloupe), OR small low-fat unsweetened banana smoothie — *<500*

Lunch: — *Calories:*

#1 **Grilled Chicken or Fish Wrap** – with banana or apple; skip the mayo & cheese. — *<500*

#2 **Salad with Grilled Chicken and Salsa** – No dressing; no croutons. — *<500*

#3 **Grilled Chicken Breast** – with steamed broccoli and ½ cup brown rice — *<500*

Dinner: — *Calories:*

#1 **6 oz. Grilled Salmon** – with whole grain pasta (1/2 c. cooked) topped with mushrooms/broccoli & tsp. olive oil — *<500*

#2 **6 oz. Grilled steak (size of your palm)** – with medium baked sweet potato (no butter) and fruit cup — *<500*

#3 **Grilled Chicken Breast** – with steamed broccoli and ½ cup brown rice — *<500*

* All meals served with unlimited water. May add unsweetened tea, diet soda, or skim milk

http://www.mobilehero.org©2012 HERO Inc.

Appendix F: Sleep Diary

	Sunday	Monday	Tuesday	Wednesday	Thursday	Friday	Saturday
Time Awoke							
How did I Sleep? 1-5 (5 best)							
How many times awoke at night							
Naps? Yes/No							
Exercise: What and how long?							
Watch TV before bed Yes/No							
Ate Before Bed Yes/No							
Time went to Bed?							
What I did to relax before bed							
What made me anxious before bed?							
What can I change?							
Did I make a change?							

Appendix G: Resources & Referrals

www.aap.org
The American Academy of Pediatrics: dedicated to the health and well-being of infants, children, adolescents and young adults

www.nichcy.org/
National Dissemination Center for Children with Disabilities operates as the nation's centralized information resource on disabilities and special education for children and youth ages birth through 21 years. It does so by collecting, organizing and disseminating current, accurate, research-based information about childhood disability and special education.

www.cdc.gov/
The Centers for Disease Control and Prevention (CDC) is a United States federal agency under the Department of Health and Human Services. It provides information to enhance health decisions, and it promotes health, injury prevention and education activities designed to improve the health of the people of the United States.

www.choosemyplate.gov/
MyPlate is part of a larger communications initiative based on *2010 Dietary Guidelines for Americans* to help consumers make better food choices. It is designed to remind Americans to eat healthfully; it is not intended to change consumer behavior alone. MyPlate illustrates the five food groups using a familiar mealtime visual, a place setting.

www.cms.gov
Centers for Medicare and Medicaid Services: Information on healthcare services, insurance enrollment and benefits for children and adults

www.dashdiet.org/
The DASH Diet is ranked by *US News and World Report* as the "Best and Healthiest Diet Plan." Endorsed by the American Heart Association and many federal programs, the DASH Diet was originally developed to lower blood pressure.

www.letsmove.gov/
Let's Move! is an initiative, launched by the First Lady, Michelle Obama, dedicated to solving the challenge of childhood obesity within a generation.

Appendix G: Resources and Referral

www.cdph.ca.gov/programs/wicworks/Pages/default.aspx
Women Infants and Children's Program, WIC, is a federally-funded health and nutrition program for women, infants, and children. WIC helps families by providing checks for buying healthy supplemental foods from WIC-authorized vendors, nutrition education, and help finding healthcare and other community services.

www.fitness.gov/
Presidents Council on Fitness Sports and Nutrition serves as a catalyst to promote good health through fitness, sports and nutrition for people of all ages, backgrounds and abilities through partnerships in national, state and local organizations, programs and initiatives.

www.healthfinder.gov/
A government website where one can find information and tools to help stay healthy. It provides some of the latest, most reliable information on a wide range of health topics selected from government and non-profit organizations.

www.webmd.com/
This website provides a plethora of information regarding healthy eating guides and plans for implementing exercise routines across all levels, as well as questions and answers.

www.heart.org/HEARTORG/
The American Heart Association site has a long list of resources for good health and good nutrition. The benefits of physical activity are solidly supported and well documented with programs designed to offer one support and encouragement. Techniques for weight management and stress management are also thoroughly presented.

www.rwjf.org/childhoodobesity/
The goal of the Robert Wood Johnson Foundation is to reverse the childhood obesity epidemic by 2015 by improving access to affordable healthy foods and increasing opportunities for physical activity in schools and communities across the nation. This website has a considerable number of publications on obesity-related research.